AF248898

Clinical Applications
of the
Acid Etch Technique

by
Richard J. Simonsen D.D.S.

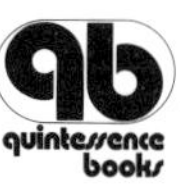

Quintessence Publishing Co., Inc. 1978
Chicago, Berlin, Rio de Janeiro, Tokyo

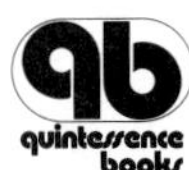

© 1978 by Quintessence Publishing Co., Inc., Chicago, Illinois.
All rights reserved.

Lithography: Industrie- und Presseklischee, Berlin
Composition: Kupijai & Prochnow, Berlin
Printing and binding: North Central Publishing Co., St. Paul
Printed in the U.S.A.

ISBN: 0–931386–01–2

Preface

The Greek philosopher *Heraclitus* once stated, "All is flux, nothing stands still." The same philosopher observed that "Nothing endures but change." These statements aptly describe not only the state of the art of dentistry, but in particular new techniques such as the acid etch technique.

It is extremely difficult to attempt description of a technique that is undergoing rapid change and prolification of uses, without becoming obsolete before getting into print. Hopefully, however, the reader will be able to grasp the magnitude of the changes the acid etch technique has already wrought on dentistry, anticipate the changes that are to come and, most importantly, open his mind to accept these changes by putting behind him the traditional narrow-mindedness that plagues the profession.

This clinically oriented book presents techniques that are sometimes radical departures from the traditionally accepted methods of practice. Many techniques described here have evolved after changing the method each time it was attempted and hopefully the reader will see that the most important aspect of the technique is the operator's willingness to accept that the only way to improve a technique is to change it.

The greatest benefit, of many that this technique offers, is the saving of tooth structure. The alternative traditional techniques invariably entail preparation of the teeth and removal of healthy enamel or dentin. With less removal of healthy tooth structure, the strength of the tooth is maintained and its lifespan increased.

Michael G. Buonocore, the father of the acid etch technique, must be gratified, indeed, to see the effect his idea is having on dentistry. The acid etch technique will undoubtedly become an even larger part of dental practice in the years to come.

Since this book is to be heavily clinically oriented, readers desiring a deeper basic knowledge of the technique than is presented here, should refer to the following excellent texts:

Adhesive Restorative Dentistry,
> *Robert L. Ibsen*
> *Kris Neville*
> W. B. Saunders Co., Philadelphia, 1974.

The Use of Adhesives in Dentistry,
> *Michael G. Buonocore*
> Charles C. Thomas, Publisher, Springfield, Illinois, 1975.

Proceedings of an International Symposium on the Acid Etch Technique. Edited by
> *Leon M. Silverstone* and
> *I. Leon Dogon*
> North Central Publishing Co., St. Paul, Minnesota, 1975.

For German readers, the following text will be of interest.

Adhäsive Zahnheilkunde
F. Lutz
B. Lüscher
H. Ochsenbein and
H. R. Mühlemann
Juris Druck & Verlag, Zürich, 1976.

One use of the acid etch technique that is not covered in the book, is the bonding of orthodontic brackets to teeth. The basic principles of bonding that are covered in the book apply also to the bonding of brackets. The other factors, such as type of brackets to use and design of the fixed appliance, belong in an orthodontic text, and not here. There is no doubt that the acid etch bonding of brackets will gain in popularity with orthodontists, (and their patients), in the future. The reader interested in the orthodontic uses of the acid etch technique is directed to the references of *Björn Zachrisson*, listed in the general reading list at the end of Chapter 10.

Some repetition of technique in the chapters is inevitable. An attempt has been made to minimize repetition. In order that some chapters can be read individually, however, without having to refer elsewhere, certain facts have been repeated.

The illustrations have been condensed down from a collection of approximately 7000 slides on the acid etch technique. Originally, 350 slides were chosen as "essential". The cost of printing color slides has necessitated almost halving this number. I am, however, extremely grateful to the publisher, Mr. *H. W. Haase*, who insisted that no sacrifice in quality was to be made when reducing the number of color illustrations to an economically feasible number. It is hoped that the selection of almost 200 color illustrations has successfully balanced cost and quality.

Acknowledgements

'Nothing is there more friendly to a man than a friend in need",
Titus Maccius Platus. 254–184 B.C.

The author extends his warmest thanks to the following friends and colleagues for their invaluable assistance in the preparation of this book.

To my colleague, *Kathleen Krenz* and dental assistants *Gail Bersie, Pam Fenner* and *Lynn Nelson* – thank you for your friendship, support and professional excellence – qualities that have been needed and much appreciated.

To my good friends at 3M Company, Dental Products Division, *Ken Allison* and *Dick Joos* in particular—thank you for your cooperation, support and technical assistance.

To *Beth Davidian* and *Laura Sweeney* at the University of Minnesota—thank you for your technical assistance with the scanning electron microscopy.

To *Fran Heille*—thank you for your invaluable and first-rate secretarial assistance and attention to detail in the preparation and typing of the manuscript.

To Dr. *Richard Chaikin* and Mr. *H. W. Haase* of Quintessence—thank you; without you both, this book would still be in my head.

Finally, to five people who have influenced the course of my personal and professional life more than any others, apart from my parents:

Jann Brevig D.D.S., in the private practice of dentistry in Tönsberg, Norway, who set me on the road to dentistry as a career.

Roy Griak, track coach at the University of Minnesota, who made it financially possible for me to come to the United States, and who was a father-figure for me during my years at the University of Minnesota.

Michael J. Till, D.D.S., M.S., Ph.D., Chairman, Department of Pedodontics, University of Minnesota, whose influence, guidance and assistance enabled me to develop my interest in pediatric dentistry to its fullest.

Leon M. Silverstone D.D.Sc., Ph.D., B.Ch.D., Professor and Head, Division of Cariology, The University of Iowa, whose inspiration and support sparked and molded my interest in the acid etch technique.

Elisabeth Magnus Simonsen, my wife, whose patience, support and love will always be needed and cherished.

Contents

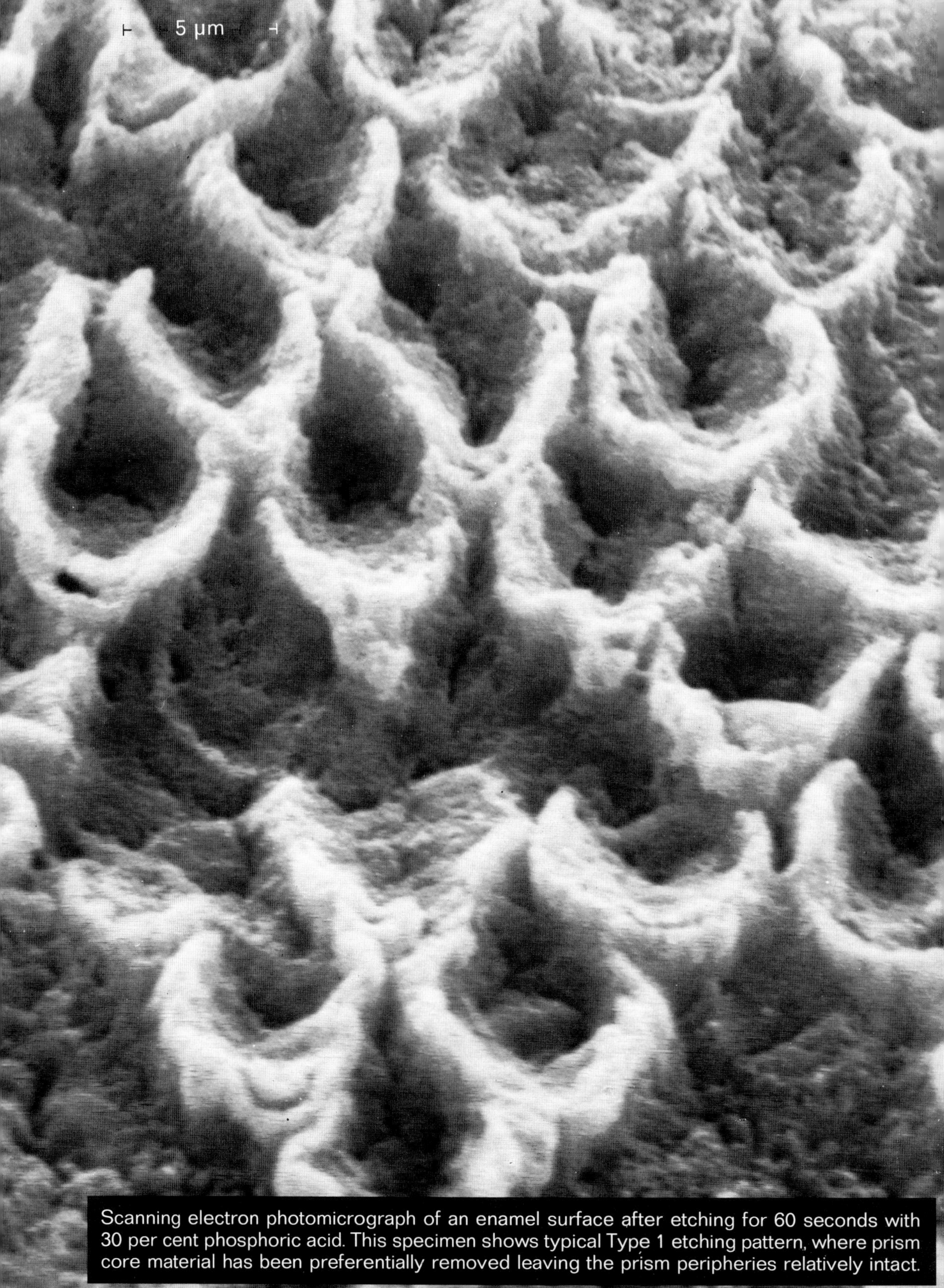

Scanning electron photomicrograph of an enamel surface after etching for 60 seconds with 30 per cent phosphoric acid. This specimen shows typical Type 1 etching pattern, where prism core material has been preferentially removed leaving the prism peripheries relatively intact.

Chapter 1

Present Status of the Acid Etch Technique

The development of the acid etch technique over the past twenty years has changed the practice of dentistry more than any other single principle recently formulated. The significance of *Michael Buonocore's* pioneering essay[1] concerning the bonding of acrylic restorative material to enamel, has not even today been recognized by more than a minority of dentists.

It took many years for others to pick up on the technique, and it has only been since 1971, when the L. D. Caulk Co. of Milford, Delaware, introduced the Nuva System of ultraviolet light activated resin, that the use of the technique has mushroomed.

Critical to the expansion in the use of the technique, was the development of the resin system (Bis-GMA) in use today in almost all commercially available composites. In 1957 the monomer was invented at the National Bureau of Standards which made composite resin restorative materials feasible. *R. L. Bowen*, who did the initial work on this resin system, (known as Bowen's formula), is still deeply involved in resin research and he deserves much credit for the present quality of the commercially available composite resins.

Improvements in etching liquids have come about in recent years largely as a result of the work of *Leon Silverstone*. Working with several acids in various strengths, *Silverstone*[8] concluded that, "unbuffered 30 per cent phosphoric acid proved to be the most satisfactory conditioning fluid ...".

Many other investigators have made significant contributions to the refinement of the materials and the technique of bonding composite resins to tooth enamel. It is, however, *Buonocore, Bowen* and *Silverstone* who stand out as the major contributors to this exciting and rapidly developing field within dentistry.

Basic Technique

The bonding of resins to enamel is effected by the mechanical retention of the material within the surface layer of enamel. This surface layer is roughened by an etching agent and the enamel prism patterns created, form a matrix into and around which the resin can flow and polymerize forming so-called "tags". These resin "tags" are the keys to the success of all acid etch bonding. Without "tags" there would be no retention and this is why the term "bonding" will be used here, rather than "adhesion".

Buonocore in his textbook "The Use of Adhesives in Dentistry",[2] delves deeply into the semantics of adhesion and bonding, and thoroughly describes the nature of adhesion. Until a material is produced that will adhere to unetched enamel, it is felt the term "bonding" better describes the attachment of resins to tooth enamel, although *Buonocore* presents a lot of evidence for his preference of the term "adhesion" to describe the same phenomenon.

Etching Agent

Buonocore[1] initially used 85 per cent phosphoric acid for his etch of enamel. This strength was apparently chosen in deference to the industrial use of phosphoric acid used in treating metal surfaces to obtain improved adhesion of paint and resin coatings.

Ten years later, *Gwinnett* and *Buonocore*[4] published the results of testing several etching agents. They reported that, "With the solutions of phosphoric acid, it was noted that with increasing concentrations progressively less change was produced on the enamel surface." The same authors later describe the effect of etching on enamel as "an increase in porosity, with the prism cores being preferentially dissolved".[5]

The most recent significant work on acid strength has been done by *Leon Silverstone*[8], who confirmed an inverse relationship between acid strength and change in surface topography on enamel, when using the acid of choice, orthophosphoric acid.

Additionally, and more importantly, *Silverstone* found that the depth of histological change was greatest at weaker acid concentrations. This area of histologically changed enamel allows the resin to form the "tags that are the foundation for the mechanical retention of the resin within the enamel." At weaker acid solutions, however, the loss in surface contour is greatest, and the ideal acid for etching combines the least loss in surface contour with the greatest depth of histologic change.

As can be seen from Figure I-1, 30 per cent H_3PO_4 produced a surface loss of 10 microns and a depth of histologic change of 20 microns, for a total depth effect of 30 microns. *Silverstone's* conclusion was that "un-

buffered 30 per cent phosphoric acid proved to be the most satisfactory conditioning fluid…" *Silverstone* also found the ideal etching time to be one minute (Fig. I-2).

Silverstone's[9] later studies confirmed his earlier results, and it has become generally accepted that etching with 30 to 40 per cent H_3PO_4 will provide the ideal surface contour for retention.

Buonocore, who developed the ultraviolet curing Nuva System of resins, still feels that 50 per cent phosphoric acid buffered with 7 per cent zinc oxide, as used with that system, is optimal. He feels that the histologic depth of the etch is less important than the number and width of pores created, into which the resin can penetrate. According to *Buonocore*, his unpublished studies suggest that there is little significant statistical difference between the etching of enamel by 30 per cent to 65 per cent phosphoric acid for 30 seconds, 60 seconds or 120 seconds.[3]

A study by *Rock*,[7] however, tends to support the use of phosphoric acid in the 30 per cent range. When comparing the bond strength of *Silverstone's* recommended 30 per cent H_3PO_4, with the more commonly used 50 per cent H_3PO_4 buffered with 7 per cent zinc oxide, *Rock* found an increase in the tensile strength of a sealant bond of over 50 per cent with the weaker acid.

Enamel is predominantly hydroxyapatite, $Ca_{10}(PO_4)_6(OH)_2$. The hydroxyapatite crystals are packed together to form prisms which, in the mature tissue, are flattened hexagons in transverse section. The prisms are oriented at right angles to the enamel surface, thus providing a latticework surface that when selectively etched produces an ideal base for the mechanical attachment of resins.

Silverstone et al[9] described three basic types of surface characteristics in etched enamel. "In the most common, called type 1 etching pattern, prism core material was preferentially removed, leaving the prism peripheres relatively intact (page 12). In the second, type 2 etching pattern, the reverse pattern was observed. The peripheral regions of prisms were removed preferentially, leaving prism cores remaining relatively unaffected. In the type 3 etching pattern, there was a more random pattern, areas of which corresponded to types 1 and 2 damage together with regions in which the pattern of etching could not be related to prism morphology."

All three etching types were found in single samples of etched enamel, suggesting that "there is no one specific etching pattern produced in human dental enamel by the actions of acid solution".

Gwinnett,[6] another knowledgeable author who has done much work on the subject, reported similar findings, "Summarily the most common appearance of the conditioned enamel surface is that of rods showing a preferred loss of material from the rod cores. Less frequently, the preferred loss is from the peripheries. Such losses are not clinically predictable and preferred loss at cores and peripheries may occur at adjacent sites in the same tooth".

The etched surface is of critical importance to the strength of the bond, for it is into this roughened surface, (page 12), that the resin flows, forming the "tags" that are the basis for retention. The surface not only must be etched for the correct time with the ideal strength of the best acid, it also must be dry and free of contaminants when the resin is applied.

Resin Material

There are two basic types of resin material on the market today; those that contain an ultraviolet catalyst and are polymerized by exposure to ultraviolet light, and those that when mixed polymerize chemically. The main advantage of the latter is the cost savings in not having to invest in an ultraviolet light; the main advantage with an ultraviolet light is that the operator has better control over the setting time.

All the resin-based materials available consist mainly of dimethacrylates or a mixture of mono- and dimethacrylate resins. Inorganic fillers, such as quartz or silica are used in the filled resin (composite) to increase strength and hardness, reduce polymerization shrinkage and increase wear resistance.

The forerunner of the ultraviolet systems was the Nuva System basically developed by *Buonocore*. Several other systems are available, including one (Alpha System, Amalgamated Dental, London), that uses a quartz fiberoptic for the delivery of the ultraviolet light, thus minimizing the size of the handpiece. Using fiberoptics also keeps the hot ultraviolet bulb away from the patient's face and minimizes scatter radiation. A disadvantage of the fiberoptic is the small area of ultraviolet light that is delivered from the handpiece, which makes polymerization of large areas more time-consuming.

The chemically curing resins have been many in number and variable in quality over the years. Because the best to emerge are basically very similar, a detailed description of one chemically curing sealant will be presented.

The Concise Enamel Bond System (3M Company, St. Paul, Minnesota) comes with both an unfilled and a filled resin, designed to be used together or independently. Basically, for fissure sealing, only the unfilled resin is used. A technique of diluting the filled resin for use as a restorative material, and at the same time a fissure sealant, is described in Chapter VIII.

The Concise Enamel Bond System uses a 37 per cent orthophosphoric acid solution (by weight), which falls within the ideal range quoted by *Silverstone*[8]. A 60 second etch time is recommended for adult enamel. The approximate surface loss of 8 to 10 microns after etching for 60 seconds can be compared to, for example, the 5 to 10 microns that are lost during a pumice prophylaxis. (Normal enamel is between 1000 and 2000 microns thick except as it tapers off towards the cervical margin.)

The Enamel Bond System consists basically of a resin from the Bowen formula; that is, the dimethacrylate addition reaction product of bisphenol A and glycidyl methacrylate. To decrease the viscosity of this resin, an active diluent, triethylene glycol dimethacrylate, is added. In an Enamel Bond kit, this resin comes in two parts, to one part a benzoyl peroxide catalyst is added, to the other an aromatic amine accelerator is added. When the two parts are mixed in equal volumes for 10 seconds there is approximately 50 seconds of working time. The resin will have a greasy appearance on polymerization, as the surface layer is inhibited from curing by oxygen in the atmosphere.

The Enamel Bond System resin will form a chemical bond with its composite filling material counterpart, Concise, because of the similarity of resin and curing agents. Most presently available filled resin systems can be used in conjunction with any unfilled resin.

Polymerization in the ultraviolet activated resins is initiated by the production of free radicals from the reaction of ultraviolet radiation with a free radical generating compound. In the self-curing or autopolymerizing systems, free radicals are generated by chemical reaction.

Clinical Applications

Initially, the acid etch technique was used purely as a means of bonding resins into the occlusal pits and fissures to prevent caries. Soon, it became evident, through the research of *Buonocore*, that another ideal area for use of the system was with the restoration of anterior fractures.

At the present time there is hardly an area of dentistry, excepting perhaps exodontics, where the acid etch technique cannot be applied. The chapters following will describe the techniques for the many uses of the system.

| | Concentration of phosphoric acid, % | | | | | | |
One minute exposure	20	30	40	50	50 ZnO	60	70
Depth of etch	14	10	9	7	6	2	2
Depth of histologic change	20	20	15	12	10	4	2
Total depth of enamel affected	34	30	24	19	16	6	4

Fig. I-1 Depth of etch and histological change in enamel (to nearest μm) following a 1-minute exposure to various concentrations of phosphoric acid. (From *Silverstone, L. M.:* Caries Res. 8:8, 1974.)

| | Concentration of phosphoric acid, % | | | | | | |
Exposure time in minutes	20	30	40	50	50 ZnO	60	70
1	14	10	9	7	6	2	2
2	17	15	14	9	7	5	2
5	40	34	27	14	11	5	2

50 ZnO = 50% phosphoric acid + 7% zinc oxide by weight

Fig. I-2 Loss in depth of surface contour (to nearest μm) after exposure to various concentrations of phosphoric acid. (From *Silverstone, L. M.:* Caries Res. 8:7, 1974.)

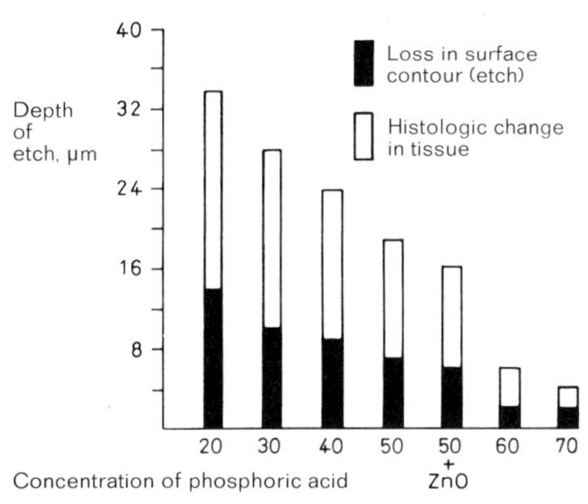

Fig. I-3 Depth of enamel affected by 1 minute exposures to various concentrations of phosphoric acid. This consists of both the loss in depth due to etching and the region showing histological change. (From *Silverstone, L. M.:* Caries Res. 8: 8, 1974.)

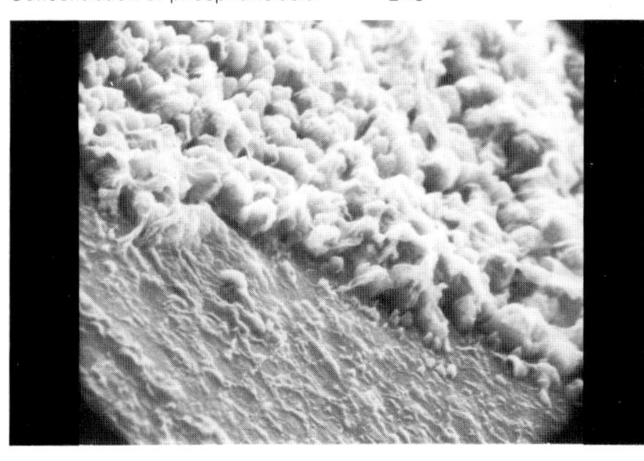

Fig. I-4 Scanning electron photomicrograph of resin base "tags". This specimen was prepared by etching part of an enamel surface with 30 per cent phosphoric acid, applying unfilled resin and then dissolving the enamel in hydrochloric acid. The margin between unetched and etched enamel, where the "tags" begin, is clearly seen.

References

1. *Buonocore, M. G.:*
   A simple method of increasing the adhesion of acrylic filling materials to enamel surfaces. J. Dent. Res. 34: 849–853, 1955.

2. *Buonocore, M. G.:*
   The Use of Adhesives in Dentistry, Charles C. Thomas Publisher, Springfield, Illinois, 1975.

3. *Buonocore, M. G.:*
   Personal Communication, 1977.

4. *Gwinnett, A. J. and Buonocore, M. G.:*
   Adhesives and caries prevention: a preliminary report. Br. Dent. J. 119: 77–80, 1965.

5. *Gwinnett, A. J. and Buonocore, M. G.:*
   A scanning electron microscope study of pit and fissure surface conditioned for adhesive sealing. Arch. Oral Biol. 17: 415–423, 1972.

6. *Gwinnett, A. J.:*
   The bonding of sealants to enamel. J. Am. Soc. Prev. Dent. 1: 21–29, 1973.

7. *Rock, W. P.:*
   The effect of etching of human enamel upon bond strengths with fissure sealant resins. Arch. Oral Biol. 19: 873–877, 1974.

8. *Silverstone, L. M.:*
   Fissure sealants: Laboratory studies. Caries Res. 8: 2–26, 1974.

9. *Silverstone, L. M., Saxton, C. A., Dogon, I. L. and Fejerskov, O.:*
   Variation in the pattern of acid etching of human dental enamel examined by scanning electron microscopy. Caries Res. 9: 373–387, 1975.

Chapter 2

Pit and Fissure Sealants

The term sealant is used to describe a resin material that is introduced into the occlusal pits and fissures of caries-susceptible teeth, thus forming a mechanical physical protective layer against the action of caries-producing bacteria and substrates.

The introduction of such materials has provided the missing link for the theoretical complete prevention of dental caries. In the past, despite diligent oral hygiene, optimal fluoride environment and adequate diet, occlusal caries was unavoidable for most people. The means to prevent occlusal caries is now here in the form of pit and fissure sealants.

The problems with pit and fissure caries were recognized long ago. *Hyatt*[12] proposed a solution to the problem in 1923 in which cavities were prepared and filled with amalgam in all pits and fissures. This was the famous "prophylactic odontotomy". There are still many practitioners active today who prefer the prophylactic odontotomy to pit and fissure sealants. This attitude seems somewhat akin to justifying suicide with the argument that death comes to everyone sooner or later in any event.

Enamel fissure eradication is also still seen occasionally. This was proposed by *Bodecker*[2, 3] as a solution to pit and fissure caries. The idea was to prepare the pits and fissures into wide rounded channels mechanically, thus eliminating the sharp food-re-tentive areas. As with *Hyatt's* prophylactic odontotomy, *Bodecker's* enamel fissure eradication involved the removal of healthy tooth structure with no guarantee that a less cariogenic situation was being created.

The incorporation of fluoride into the drinking water supplies of cities has, over the years, had a tremendous effect on reducing the incidence of caries. Studies, such as the one of *Ast* et al.[1] have reported significant drops of 50 to 60 per cent in the caries rates of children of various ages.

It is generally accepted, that the beneficial effect of either ingested or topically applied fluoride is in prevention and control of smooth-surface caries. With ideal fluoride environment, it is suspected that pit and fissure caries is delayed one or two years, but it is certainly not prevented on the scale that smooth-surface caries is. Pit and fissure sealing, therefore, can have a tremendous impact on caries incidence.

Technique for fissure sealing

The basic technique for fissure sealing follows. Variations do occur, particularly in methods of isolation, but the step-by-step procedure for etching and sealing is a simple process that can be quickly learned by dentist, hygienist or assistant. The important point to be remembered is that the success of sealant retention is totally technique dependent. As soon as the operator has mastered the technique and adheres strictly to the principles of sealant application, sealant retention will be almost 100%. Only in cases where the technique has broken down (such as with salivary contamination of the etched surface), will there be sealant loss. It cannot be emphasized enough, that meticulous attention to the details of the technique, will lead to rewarding experiences when recalling patients for checking sealant retention.

Step 1. Selection of patients and teeth

As with any technique, pit and fissure sealing is not indicated for every child. In cases where rampant or moderate decay exists and the chances for interproximal decay are high, one does not save very much by placing sealant on occlusal pits and fissures. Similarly, there are those patients with no clinical caries and coalesced fissures, (shallow, rounded grooves), where caries is extremely unlikely. Again, in such cases, applying sealant is a waste of the operator's, and the patient's, time.

Many children, however, have occlusal anatomy that experience tells us will surely lead to decay within 6 months or one year (Figs. II-5 and II-15). These children with sharp, deep pits and fissures, with possibly evidence of previous occlusal caries (Fig. II-5) are prime candidates for sealant application. It is just physically impossible to clean out the deep fissure anatomy on most children's teeth. The tooth brush bristle is much too wide to penetrate into the average occlusal groove. Thus, even though the child may have a good diet, excellent oral hygiene, regular dental visits and optimal fluoride environment, occlusal caries is still inevitable in most children.

Step 2. Cleaning the teeth

The tooth surface to be etched and sealed must be thoroughly cleaned. A pointed

bristle brush is excellent for gross plaque removal. It can be used with a pumice/water slurry, or it can be used dry. Oil-based mixtures of pumice should be avoided, as the oils may stick to the enamel surface and interfere with etching. After cleaning the occlusal pits and fissures with a pointed brush, it is good policy to drag an explorer tine through all the grooves. This will remove some of the deeper plaque that the brush cannot reach. The tooth should then be washed with water.

Step 3. Isolation

Isolation is extremely important and is probably the most critical step with regard to the success or failure of the sealant. Rubber dam is ideal for isolation. Cotton rolls, however, are more practical and much more frequently used. It is perfectly possible, with good technique, to get excellent isolation with cotton rolls and this method is recommended from a practical and cost-effective standpoint. It is estimated from the 500 patients sealed in a clinical study by the author, that isolation would have been significantly improved with use of the rubber dam in less than 5% of the cases. In these cases, however, rubber dam was essential for successful sealant application.

The use of cotton rolls for isolation requires a special technique, that once mastered, provides for a rapid and effective means of moisture control.

Mandibular right quadrant: Two cotton rolls are used initially, one lingually held down by the thumb of the operator's left hand and one buccally held down by the operator's index finger. In this way, the operator has far better control over the patient's tongue, than if a cotton roll holder was used. After etching, and washing, the cotton rolls will be saturated, and the critical moment in the technique is reached. Before drying the etched tooth, new cotton rolls are placed on top of the saturated ones which are then pulled out from under the fresh cotton roll (or sometimes the saturated roll is just left in place underneath). In this way, the operator's thumb and index finger are always in complete control of the patient's tongue and cheek. If cotton roll holders are used, there is a far greater chance of contamination during removal and exchange of the cotton rolls and holder. Care must be taken at all times to avoid salivary contamination of etched enamel. One area that is frequently neglected, is the buccal groove on mandibular first permanent molars. It is easy, during exchange of cotton rolls, to let the cheek collapse onto the buccal surface of the tooth, thus contaminating this surface. Special care must be taken when replacing the buccal cotton roll.

Two fresh cotton rolls, one on top of the other, are sometimes required lingually for patients with a heavy salivary flow. After exchange of cotton rolls, the tooth can be dried and the sealant applied.

Mandibular left quadrant: From personal preference, it is recommended to operate in this quadrant left-handed. This means the operator's right thumb is used on the lingual cotton roll and right index finger on the buccal cotton roll. One can easily adapt to completing the etching, washing and sealant application left-handed. The operator has far better control of the cotton rolls, (and it is much less strain on the wrist), using one's right hand, when sitting in the normal position for a right-handed operator.

Maxillary right quadrant: The operator's left index finger holds the buccal cotton roll in place, while the second finger is used as a guard to prevent the tongue from contaminating the lingual surfaces.

Maxillary left quadrant: The operator's second finger controls the buccal cotton roll while the index finger controls the tongue.

Step 4. Etching

After isolation, the teeth are thoroughly dried to remove any viscous saliva that may hinder acid coverage of the enamel, and the phosphoric acid is applied to the whole occlusal surface and any lingual or buccal surface where grooves require sealing. Acid can be applied with either a cotton pellet or a mini-sponge. A lockable cotton pliers is a great help to hold the pellet or sponge. The mini-sponges are excellent (Fig. II-31), for acid application and come supplied with 3M Enamel Bond or 3M White Sealant kits. As soon as the complete area to be etched is covered with acid, the time is noted, and the tooth enamel is etched for 60 seconds. Fresh acid should be continually dabbed on the surfaces to be etched, to ensure circulation of fresh acid to the enamel surface at all times. Care must be taken as the etching time progresses, to treat the enamel surface very carefully, and not rub the cotton pellet or sponge on the surface during acid application, as this may damage the fragile enamel latticework being formed. It was *Rock's*[15] impression that "bond strength was more related to the nature of the adhered surface than to the resin used".

Step 5. Washing

Another critically important step to the success or failure of the technique, is the washing-off of the phosphoric acid after etching. All too frequently this step is completed in a very cursory manner. It is imperative to remove all the phosphoric acid and the reaction precipitates produced during etching. For this, water under pressure and a water-air spray is essential, along with high power evacuation.

Initially, pure water is used to remove most of the acid. The evacuator tip should be placed adjacent to the tooth and the water directed towards the tip. In this way, one retards saturation of the cotton rolls, thereby minimizing the chances for the overflow of saliva onto the etched surface. After approximately 5 seconds of pure water, the air button is also pressed forming a strong water-spray which should be played over the etched surface for at least 15–20 seconds. An etched tooth cannot be satisfactorily washed over all surfaces in just 5–10 seconds. A minimum of 20 seconds per tooth, or 40 seconds per quadrant, is recommended. The operator should be especially aware to point the spray directly at surfaces that may be behind cusps, or otherwise out of the path of the spray (e. g. buccal and lingual surfaces).

After completion of the washing phase, the assistant removes all the excess water and saliva with the aspirator. It has been suggested by *Ibsen* and *Neville*[13] that after etching the patient should rinse, although in the same book the authors stress "isolation to prevent contamination". How these factors, (that is, rinsing and noncontamination), are compatible is hard to understand. Most authors presently agree that rinsing by the patient after etching should definitely not be allowed, and that the sealant should be applied as soon as possible after etching, washing and drying with air that is not contaminated by oil or water.

Step 6. Re-isolation

After washing of the etched surfaces, the cotton rolls will need replacing, as described previously in Step 3. If there is any salivary contamination of the etched enamel at this time, the area should be re-etched for about 10 seconds, before washing again.

Step 7. Drying the etched enamel and mixing the resin

As soon as the cotton rolls are replaced, compressed air is directed over all etched surfaces. The drying phase is also most important, as moisture on the etched surface will hinder penetration of the resin into the enamel. While the assistant is mixing or preparing the resin according to the manufacturer's instructions, air is continually directed over the etched enamel right up until the sealant is applied. A minimum of 15 seconds drying time is recommended for a single tooth and 25 seconds for a quadrant.

The air hose used for drying etched surfaces should be periodically checked, to be certain it is free of contaminants such as oil and water. Water leaking into the air hose will render the drying phase, and thus also the technique, a failure.

Step 8. Sealant Application

A brush is undoubtedly the best method of applying sealant to an etched surface. It is possible to pick up sealant with certain small metal instruments, but touching the fragile etched surface may result in damage to the etched prisms. With the ultraviolet curing systems, a brush can be used many times over. The autopolymerizing systems, however, must use disposable brushes, as it is not possible to completely remove all the resin from the bristles prior to polymerization, and after a few applications, the brush becomes clogged with resin and must be discarded.

Several brush types are pictured in Figure II-32. The top brush is a prototype of one to be marketed by the 3M Company. The whole brush (handle included) is disposable. The pointed tip at the opposite end of the brush is very useful for sealant application in areas of difficult access, where just a small drop of sealant is required (Fig. II-18). The L. D. Caulk brush, (bottom), supplied with their new filled Nuva-Cote sealant, has a disposable tip on a very nicely designed handle. The middle brush is supplied with the AlphaSeal kit, (Amalgamated Dental, London, England). It consists of a metal handle with a removable sable brush.

The sponges supplied with the 3M White Sealant, and originally intended for sealant application, are not recommended (Fig. II-31). The sponges rapidly become saturated with resin, which cannot then be extracted from the sponge without compressing the sponge on the delicate enamel surface. This is definitely contraindicated. In addition to possibly damaging the fragile enamel surface, the use of sponges tends to increase the number of bubbles within the sealant.

Delton Pit and Fissure Sealant (Johnson and Johnson, East Windsor, New Jersey) has a unique applicator, consisting of disposable plastic tubes into which sealant is drawn up by suction. The end of the tube is then placed on the tooth and the sealant expelled. The idea behind this principle is excellent, but the size of the tube makes delicate application in difficult areas (close to gingiva or areas of restricted access) a problem.

Sealant should be applied in a relatively thick layer (Fig. II-6). It is better to apply too much, which may cause a temporary occlusal interference until the high-spot is rapidly abraded away by the forces of mastication, (probably within 24 hours), than to apply too little. The thicker the sealant, the longer it will last. A thin layer of sealant may not have the strength to resist fracture.

When applying autopolymerizing sealant to a whole quadrant, it is best to cover all the etched areas on each tooth as soon as possible with a layer of sealant, and then go back to each tooth and add bulk as necessary. This is done to ensure that fresh resin is used to cover the etched enamel for optimal "tag" penetration. Should insufficient sealant have been mixed initially, fresh unpolymerized resin can always be mixed and added to the polymerized material provided isolation has been maintained.

Most sealants polymerize in 1–3 minutes. The outer surface layer of any sealant will not polymerize, due to the inhibiting effect of the oxygen in the atmosphere on the reaction. Thus the sealant will always appear to have a greasy film after polymerization. This film should be wiped off, so as to minimize the unpleasant taste of resin in the patient's mouth.

The complete procedure from Step 3, after isolation of a quadrant, to polymerization of the sealant, should take approximately 3½ minutes. Assuming one applies sealant to only one quadrant at a time, a patient should be able to have four quadrants sealed in less than 20 minutes from seating to dismissal. The average times, in the 3M White Sealant study to be discussed later in this chapter, for four quadrant application was 19 minutes, and for four single tooth (first permanent molars) quadrants was 15 minutes. The breakdown of one quadrant is approximately:

Etch	60 seconds
Wash	30 seconds
Change cotton rolls Dry tooth Mix sealant	30 seconds
Apply sealant	30 seconds
Polymerization	60 seconds
Total time	3½ minutes

Indications for Use of Sealants

1. Deep pits and fissures on molars (or bicuspids) that are likely to become carious.
2. Minimal or questionable fissure caries. Technique described in Chapter VIII.
3. Patient is unable to maintain ideal oral hygiene (handicapped child).

Contraindications to Use of Sealants

1. Rampant or moderate decay where interproximal caries is probable in the future.
2. Rounded, shallow fissures where decay is unlikely.

Questions frequently raised concerning sealants and the acid etch technique

1. What happens to etched areas that are not covered by sealant?

The areas of etched enamel not covered by resin, return to their original appearance and approach the same levels of acid resistance as adjacent unetched enamel within 24 hours, *Silverstone*.[18] Remineralization, by deposition of the organic and mineral components of saliva, and fluoride, (from drinking water or other sources), account for this rapid return to normalcy.

2. Why does a stronger solution of phosphoric acid create a less desirable etching pattern than a weaker solution?

This question is still unanswered. *Silverstone*[17] has suggested that it "may be related to the degree of ionization of the acid. The weaker the acid the greater the ionization, and therefore the greater effect of diffusion into the tissue. In addition, one must consider the formation of other phases, in this way soluble or insoluble precipitates will affect further the dissolution rate".

3. Does spillage of phosphoric acid onto soft tissue create any undesirable effect?

It is a frequent occurrence for the etching agent to contact soft tissue during etching for sealant application, particularly in areas adjacent to buccal and lingual grooves. No adverse reaction has ever been seen or documented from phosphoric acid acting on the gingiva or oral mucosa for short periods of time.

4. What happens if a carious lesion is inadvertently sealed over?

Studies by *Handelman*[10] indicate that sealing over diagnosed carious lesions results in a decrease in the viable bacteria count (a 2000-fold decrease after 2 years). Preliminary clinical and radiographic findings suggest that there was no progression of the carious lesions.

It is still not presently recommended to deliberately seal over carious lesions. *Handelman's* studies, however, indicate that there is no cause for concern over the inadvertant sealing-over of undetectable dental caries.

5. A related question is, can caries be initiated under a sealant?

Properly applied sealants do not leak and thus the initiation of decay is not possible. Figures II-33 and 34 show SEM views of a sealant after 18 months in the mouth. Close examination all around the margins of this, and several other specimens, has never revealed any sign of leaky margins. The case seen in Figures II-28 to 30 shows the only example of a leaky margin seen clinically in over 2700 teeth sealed. It is feasible that caries could initiate below a margin that has "lifted" and is leaking. This is not the fault of the material, however, for some error in technique, (possibly the groove was subgingival at application and did not etch properly, or the etched enamel was contaminated by the capillary action of adjacent tissue fluids), was responsible for the margin leaking. The question of whether the sealant, in such a case, can contribute to caries initiation becomes academic when one considers that only the most caries-susceptible teeth are sealed in the first place.

6. What happens to the maturation of enamel after sealant application immediately posteruption?

If maturation of enamel is defined as the acquisition of organic and inorganic material by immature enamel, then the application of resin would stop maturation of sealed enamel. The basic question is, however, at just what stage after eruption can maturation be said to have reached an optimal level? In vitro studies by *Silverstone*,[19] simulating posteruptive maturation of enamel, show no additional benefit to the surface enamel after 48 hours of exposure to the oral fluids. If maturation is a protective process that continues for some time after eruption, it apparently does little to protect against pit and fissure caries, which can frequently be diagnosed before a tooth is even fully erupted. Thus application of a sealant to a caries-sus ceptible fissure can certainly not have a deleterious effect on the tooth if it prevents caries at the expense of the maturation of the sub-sealant enamel.

7. How long will sealants last?

This probably is the most frequently asked question by parents, and it is the hardest to answer. *Buonocore*[4] expects properly applied sealants to show a half-life of approximately four years. *Horowitz*[11] has presented the 5-year results of the Kalispell study, which showed that 42% of the teeth examined at 5 years still retained all the sealant, 14% had sealant partially missing and 44% had no visibly retained sealant. With improvements in materials and techniques, it is hoped that the 5-year retention figures will be dramatically improved. Possibly a 90% retention figure at 5 years is not an unrealistic goal.

8. Can partially lost sealants increase the chance of caries developing?

Horowitz,[11] reported in his 5-year Kalispell results, that 7% of the teeth with sealant partially missing became carious, whereas comparison with that group's paired, unsealed controls, showed a 41% caries incidence. One cannot preclude the possibility that in the group of 7% with sealant partially missing that became carious, are some teeth that decayed as a result of the partially missing sealant creating a cariogenic situation. However, it is clear from *Horowitz's* results, that even partially sealed teeth are considerably less susceptible to decay, than unsealed teeth.

Charbeneau,[5] in a recently published study, concluded that "Sealant loss from a surface did not appear to initiate pit and fissure caries on maxillary teeth. Such loss may have been a contributing factor in 6 of 38 mandibular tooth surfaces".

9. Can amalgams be covered with sealant?

There is no adhesion or bonding between silver amalgam and sealant resin. However, in the case of small, single-surface amalgams, marginal leakage of the amalgam can be eliminated, (and thus secondary caries potential eliminated), if the amalgam is covered with a layer of sealant.

If, during a routine sealant appointment, small amalgams, such as that seen in Figure II-13, are seen, it certainly will not do any harm to cover them up (Fig. II-14). It is assumed that there is no clinically or roentgenographically diagnosable caries associated with the amalgam. The life of the amalgam will be extended for as long as the sealant is covering all the amalgam margins. Even when the sealant wears down to the amalgam surface, such as will soon be the case in Figure II-12, where the sealant has been covering an occlusal amalgam for 12 months, the marginal leakage of the amalgam will still be less than it would be with no sealant present, since sealant is present between the amalgam and enamel walls.

It must be remembered when sealing over amalgams, as the amalgam increases in size, so the sealant retentive area decreases. Thus, it would not be recommended to seal-over amalgams larger than those seen in Figure II-25.

10. Can dental auxiliaries apply sealant?

Each state legislates the scope of practice of dentists and auxiliaries alike. A properly trained auxiliary can be just as successful at sealant application as a dentist. In a study by *Stiles,*[22] it was observed that there was "no difference in the retention of the sealant when applied by a dentist or a trained dental auxiliary ...".

Increasing use of dental auxiliaries should enable more children to be sealed for less cost. Provided proper training and supervision is given, there is no reason why dentists should object to expanding the role of dental auxiliaries to include the application of pit and fissure sealant.

Problems encountered during sealant application

The tremendous benefits of adding color to sealants, (the first colored sealant on the market was the 3M Concise Brand White Sealant System, March 1977) are clearly seen in the illustrations accompanying this chapter. The color addition also has positive side effects inasmuch as problems with sealant handling can also be documented. These problems are by no means unique to colored sealant, as they frequently may have gone unnoticed with the clear sealants.

1. Excess sealant spillage onto gingival tissues

Figure II-23 shows what can happen distal to upper molars during sealant application with the patient in the supine position. The flow of the material is to the distal, and it may, once it touches the gingiva, flow in excess onto an adjacent area. Similarly, in the buccal groove of lower molars, one frequently has to apply sealant very close to gingival tissue. Contact with the tissue will result in an excessive amount of sealant accumulating at the gingival margin.

It is best in cases such as this, to simply let the material polymerize, and then trim the material down. Trying to remove the material prior to polymerization, or attempting to flick off the excess after polymerization, may weaken the sealant bond. A 7901 FG Midwest American carbide composite finishing bur (Fig. V-5) is excellent for high-speed removal of sealant flash, leaving a relatively smooth resin surface after removal. The bur is thin enough to be able to enter the gingival sulcus without damaging the tissue.

2. Bubbles

Air bubbles within resins have always been a problem. With the introduction of colored sealant, bubbles have been more easily observed. Figure II-24 shows a maxillary first permanent molar, at the 12-month recall with a bubble apparent in the mesial portion of the sealant. This particular bubble is not of concern, but obviously it is not desirable to have sealant surfaces full of bubbles. If the bubble penetrates to the depth of the fissure or is seen to be in a potentially weak area of the sealant, another mix of sealant should be made and the bubble simply filled in. Careful instruction of the dental assistant in slow, deliberate mixing of the two resins together rather than using a rapid stirring action, will almost completely eliminate bubbles of any consequence. The 3M minisponges also have a tendency to increase the incidence of bubbles if used for resin application. As stated previously, these sponges are contraindicated for sealant application.

Reapplication of sealant

Sealant loss, if the operator follows the technique meticulously, is rare, and usually confined to areas:

1. Of difficult access (Cause: improper cleaning, etching and washing).
2. Adjacent to gingival margins (Cause: contamination by capillary action of tissue and crevicular fluids).
3. Of saliva contamination after etching (Cause: moisture control problems).

Most sealant loss, as a result of the problems noted above, will occur within the first 12 months after application. In the 3M White Sealant study to be reported here, all sealant loss was confined to the lingual of maxillary molars and the buccal of mandibular molars.

To reapply the sealant, the reason for loss should first be established, so that the error is not repeated. In the case of sealant loss soon after application, it is unlikely that the sealant penetrated the enamel to form "tags", and the enamel, after cleaning, should be just as easily etched as fresh enamel. The adjacent sealant, to which the new sealant will also bond, should have the surface layer removed with a bur to expose uncontaminated resin. In the case of sealant loss as a result of gradual abrasion, the enamel surface is probably impregnated with resin and may require a slightly increased etching time, before adding fresh resin. Figures II-27 to 30, show two cases of sealant loss, and one case of re-application.

Clinical study with 3M White Sealant

Simonsen[19] reported the first results utilizing a colored sealant.

The benefits of using a colored sealant are many. The other presently available pit and fissure sealants, (apart from the filled sealant from Kerr and Caulk's new Nuva-Cote), are all clear resins (Fig. II-2). As time progresses, these resins become increasingly difficult to detect. Adding color to the resin makes application much easier, and after polymerization the operator has no doubt that the resin is present in the amount desired. Recall examination, and tabulation of accurate retention records, are also much simplified with a colored sealant.

The question of patient and parental acceptance was one that had to be answered. Surprisingly, perhaps, there was no problem at all on this front. In fact, a benefit of the colored sealant, is that it enables the parent to see that something has actually been done. Also, it gives the child a visible motivational factor to remind him that he must keep up his part of the preventive program with brushing and flossing.

Advantages of colored sealant over clear sealant

1. Easier to apply.
2. Easier to check for complete coverage and polymerization.
3. Easier and quicker to check for retention at recall.
4. Allows more accurate tabulation of retention progress.
5. Helpful motivational agent in the overall preventive dental health program.

Material

The 3M White Sealant is a diluted Bis-GMA resin, of the autopolymerizing kind. The sealant consists basically of the clear 3M Enamel Bond resin to which has been added 2–3% submicron silica, 5–6% colloidal silica (diluted to 2–3%) and 1% Titanium Dioxide (the white coloring agent).

In initial studies with coloring agents, *Dogon* has done much unpublished work with a red pigmented Enamel Bond with excellent results. A yellow pigment was also added to Enamel Bond (Fig. II-3) before the white color was chosen. Figure II-4 shows the first white color used, a 0.5% Titanium Dioxide addition, alongside the presently used color, a 1% Titanium Dioxide addition. In this particular case, the 0.5% sealant has been bonded to the first molar for 18 months, while the 1% sealant has been bonded to the second molar for 12 months. The excellent buccal retention in both cases should be observed. Sealant application was as per the technique previously described with cotton roll isolation.

Results

The 3M White Sealant exhibits excellent retentive properties, as can be seen from Figures II-7 to 11. Even buccal and lingual retention is excellent. Of 651 buccal and lingual surfaces sealed (398 maxillary lingual and 253 mandibular buccal), only 19 surfaces showed partial loss of sealant at 6 months for a retention rate of 95.2%. At 12 months, of 213 maxillary lingual and 135 mandibular buccal surfaces, 27 showed partial loss, (or had been re-sealed at 6 months due to partial loss), for a retention rate of 92.2%. These retention rates, 95.2% at 6 months and 92.2% for

12 months, are for the most loss-prone surfaces. Retention was 99.8% for occlusal surfaces of 1709 permanent and deciduous teeth examined at 6 months, (one permanent occlusal surface and 2 deciduous occlusal surfaces were partially missing) and 99.7% for occlusal surfaces of 1019 permanent and deciduous teeth examined at 12 months, (three surfaces partially missing).
The buccal and lingual retention results would tend to question the conclusion of Cons[7] who stated that "… we would not recommend sealing the buccal groove (of mandibular molars) because the retention rate (2.7%) was low …". Once again, it should be emphasized that sealant retention is technique dependent. If thorough attention is paid to scrupulous cleaning, etching and washing after etching, of buccal and lingual grooves, the retention rates will be excellent.

Retention of 3M Concise Brand White Sealant System

6 Months After Application

Teeth	No. of Teeth Sealant Applied	No. and Retained %	No. and Partially Missing %	Totally Missing %
Permanent	1027	1011 (98.4%)	16 (1.6%)	0
Deciduous	682	678 (99.4%)	4 (0.6%)	0

Total number of patients: 265

Of the 16 teeth showing partial sealant loss at 6 months; 8 were maxillary right first molars with partial sealant loss on the lingual (as in Fig. II-29); 7 were mandibular first molars with partial sealant loss on the buccal (as in Fig. II-27); and 1 upper bicuspid showed partial loss of sealant from the occlusal surface.
Five deciduous teeth were dropped from the study at 6 months due to interproximal decay and 3 deciduous teeth exfoliated prior to the 6-month recall.

Retention of 3M Concise Brand White Sealant System

12 Months After Application

Teeth	No. of Teeth Sealant Applied	No. and Retained %	No. and Partially Missing %	Totally Missing %
Permanent	583	560 (96.1%)	23 (3.9%)	0
Deciduous	436	431 (98.9%)	5 (1.1%)	0

Total number of patients: 153

Of the 23 permanent teeth showing partial sealant loss at 12 months, 13 were cases reapplied at 6 months and present at 12 months (although obviously for study purposes counted as missing). Of the remaining 10 teeth, 6 were maxillary first molars with partial lingual sealant loss, and 4 were mandibular first molars with partial buccal sealant loss.
A further 4 deciduous teeth exfoliated prior to the 12-month recall.

Distribution of Sealed Permanent Teeth

	6 Months		12 Months	
	Total	%	Total	%
Mandibular First Molars	331	32.2	193	33.1
Maxillary First Molars	327	31.8	184	31.6
Permanent First Molar Total	658	64.0	377	64.7
Mandibular Bicuspids	151	14.7	83	14.2
Maxillary Bicuspids	143	13.9	86	14.8
Bicuspid Total	294	28.6	169	29.0
Mandibular Second Molars	40	3.9	21	3.6
Maxillary Second Molars	35	3.4	16	2.7
Permanent Second Molar Total	75	7.3	37	6.3

Patient Age at Sealing

6–Month Recall				12–Month Recall			
3 years	5%	9 years	11%	3 years	3%	9 years	15%
4 years	5%	10 years	11%	4 years	6%	10 years	5%
5 years	6%	11 years	10%	5 years	10%	11 years	10%
6 years	9%	12 years	5%	6 years	10%	12 years	6%
7 years	16%	12+ years	6%	7 years	17%	12+ years	5%
8 years	16%			8 years	13%		

Variable etch time on deciduous molars

Deciduous enamel has been described as "prismless" by *Gwinnett*.[8] *Silverstone*[19] found that only 17% of deciduous enamel could be classified as "prismless", and this was found only in the cervical regions. There is no evidence of "prismless" enamel (which requires a longer etching time for adequate etching pattern) on occlusal surfaces, yet the present recommendation for etching deciduous enamel is to double the etch time to 120 seconds, rather than utilize the 60 seconds used for permanent enamel.

To test the clinical significance of the two-minute etch time for deciduous tooth sealant retention, the etch time was varied on different quadrants in the same patient. By etching, for example, the maxillary left and mandibular right quadrants for 120 seconds, and the maxillary right and mandibular left quadrants for 60 seconds, opposite quadrants, (both left/right and up/down), were differentially etched.

Results:

No significant difference was found in the retention of sealant on teeth etched for 60 seconds or 120 seconds either at 6 months or 12 months. It appears, despite in vitro studies that show a 120-second etch is necessary for an adequate etching pattern on deciduous enamel, that this finding is not clinically significant for occlusal sealants.

It is interesting to note that at 12 months, more sealant was lost on teeth etched for 120 seconds than on teeth etched for 60 seconds. It might have been anticipated that more "failures" would occur in the 60-second etch group.

In very young children, it is frequently much more difficult to maintain adequate isolation throughout the procedure. Obviously, when etching for 120 seconds, there is a much greater chance of salivary contamination during etching, than when etching for only half that time. Two minutes with a mouthful of cotton rolls can be a long time for a three year-old child. Thus, despite the amount of sealant loss not being signif-icant to draw any conclusion as to one etch time being better than the other, it is significant that all "failures", were noted at the time of application, as being on patients where moisture control was a problem. Since a 60-second etch time appears adequate for retention, perhaps on these "failure" cases, the sealant could have been applied prior to any salivary contamination of the etched enamel, had a 60-second etch time been utilized. While rubber dam isolation is the ideal, and would ease application in certain cases, these results do not indicate that appreciable benefits in retention can be expected with use of the rubber dam as a routine method of isolation.

Deciduous Molar Retention with Variable Etch Time

6 Months

	Teeth Etched 1 minute	Teeth Etched 2 minutes	Total
	365	317	682
Partially Missing:	2	2	4
Total Retention:	99.5%	99.4%	99.4%

12 Months

	Teeth Etched 1 minute	Teeth Etched 2 minutes	Total
	183	253	436
Partially Missing:	1	4	5
Total Retention:	99.5%	98.4%	98.9%

The future for pit and fissure sealants

There is no doubt that pit and fissure sealants are here to stay. Whether they ever can be used as a mass public health measure will largely depend on cost-effectiveness studies that are under way.

The addition of fluoride to pit and fissure sealants is certainly feasible[23] and does not result in any loss of retentive quality in the sealant.[20] However, it seems somewhat academic to study the addition of fluoride to sealants if we can obtain around 90–95% sealant retention. The potential benefit is small, and how much effect would the fluoride have deep in the enamel fissure, where an organic plug prevents penetration of the sealant?

Fluoride pre-treatment of the etched enamel surface has also been studied.[6, 9, 14]

An idea this author has been studying for some time in the feasibility of interproximal sealing (Fig. II-35). There is certainly a vast potential for caries prevention. The sealant could be somewhat flexible and semi-permanent, or temporary in conjunction with a fluoride-containing sealant, or a fluoride pre-treatment of etched enamel.

The secondary preventive effect of sealants is an interesting hypothesis. It is clear from data being assembled at this time, that the patients returning for recall visits who have had all carious pits and fissures sealed, have a considerably lower incidence of interproximal caries than their unsealed peers.

This lower caries incidence may be due to several factors, including the secondary effect of motivation (to brush and floss) provided by the presence of colored sealant. Another reason may be that the original sealant population was part of a select group (selection criteria p. 20).

The role of *Streptococcus mutans in* dental caries is one that has been given much attention in dental microbiological research in recent years. The occlusal pits and fissures are a major site of *S. mutans* colonization. By blocking off this ecological niche with pit and fissure sealants one might predict a decrease in the numbers of *S. mutans* in the mouth.[16] If this is so, the incidence of dental caries may well be reduced, both directly and indirectly, by pit and fissure sealants.

Whichever direction sealant research is to take, it is an exciting field, full of challenges for the years to come.

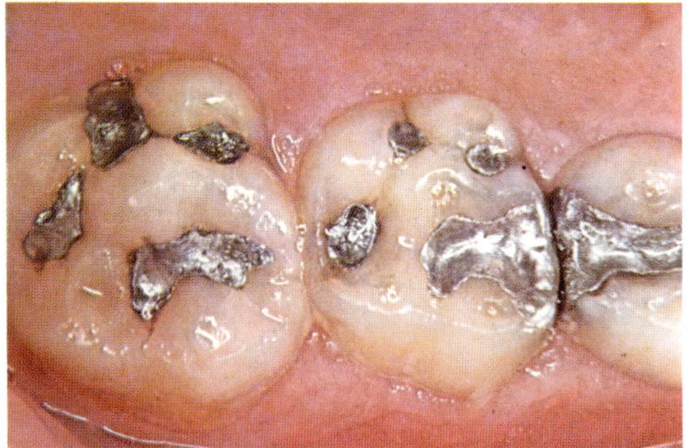

Fig. II-1   Patient N. W. The first permanent molar in this young child has already four separate amalgam restorations. Unrestored grooves and poor amalgam margins predispose to secondary caries attack. The application of pit and fissure sealants at an early age can frequently eliminate the need for multiple restorations and prevent secondary caries.

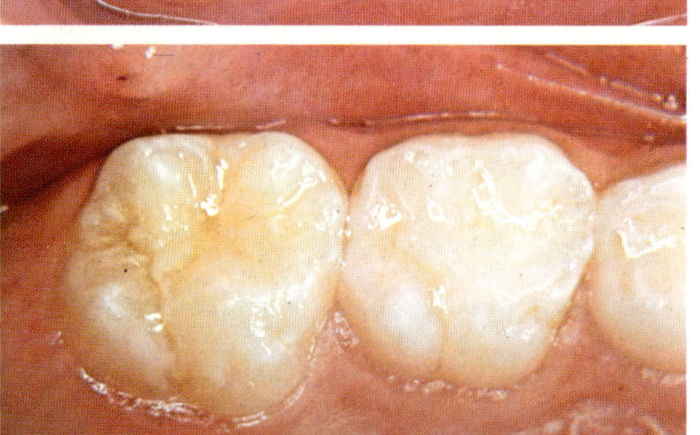

Fig. II-2   Patient K. S. The first pit and fissure sealants introduced were all clear resins similar to the 3M Enamel Bond seen here immediately after application. The light reflection discloses the presence of the shiny newly applied sealant, but after some months in the mouth it becomes increasingly difficult to detect the presence of clear sealants.

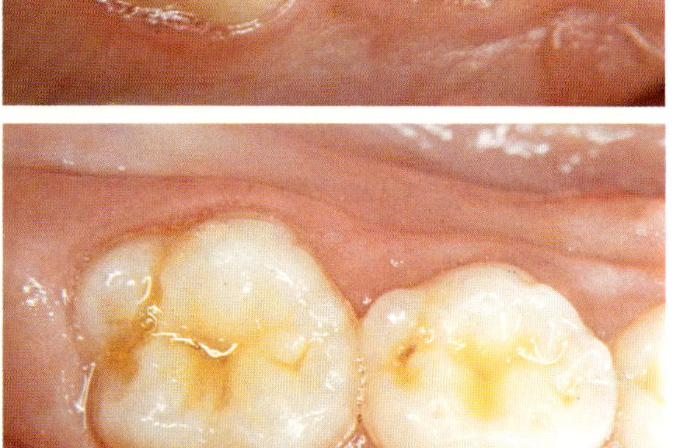

Fig. II-3   Patient M. M. In the first clinical trials with colored sealant, several colors (yellow, red and white) were tested. This patient was treated with a yellow Enamel Bond which, as this 6-month recall case demonstrates, was retained well and was clearly visible on recall.

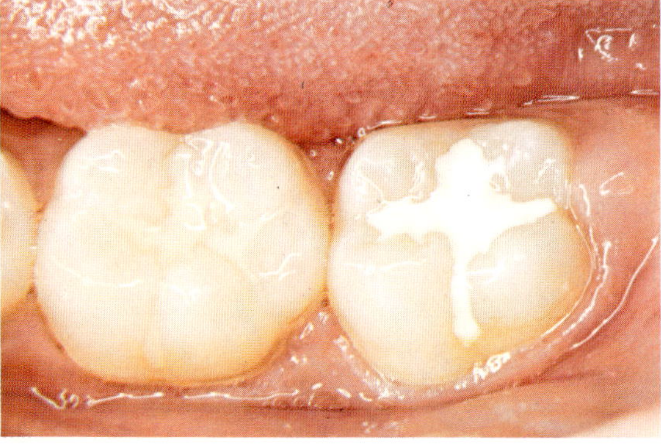

Fig. II-4   Patient J. G. Two different strengths of white color were also tested. The lighter white color as seen on this lower first permanent molar, became sometimes a little difficult to distinguish from the natural tooth color, whereas the stronger white was always clearly visible. Note the excellent retention, even buccally, for both the light sealant (18 months after application) and the bright sealant (12 months after application).

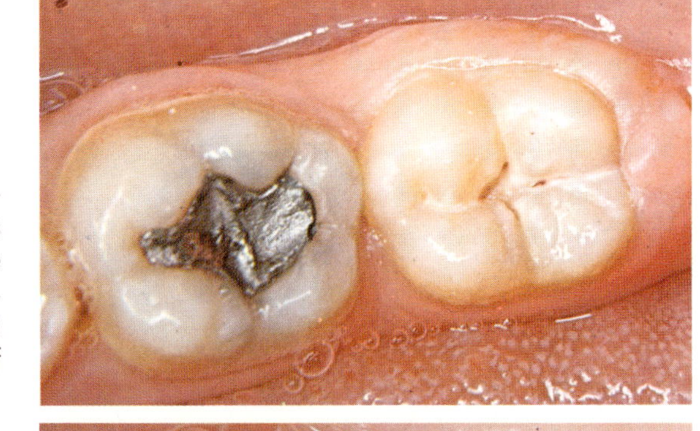

Fig. II-5 Patient K. B. It does not take much foresight to predict that the occlusal surface of this second permanent molar will very soon become carious. If careful clinical and radiographic examination fails to diagnose caries, such teeth should be sealed immediately after thorough cleaning of the deeply grooved occlusal surface.

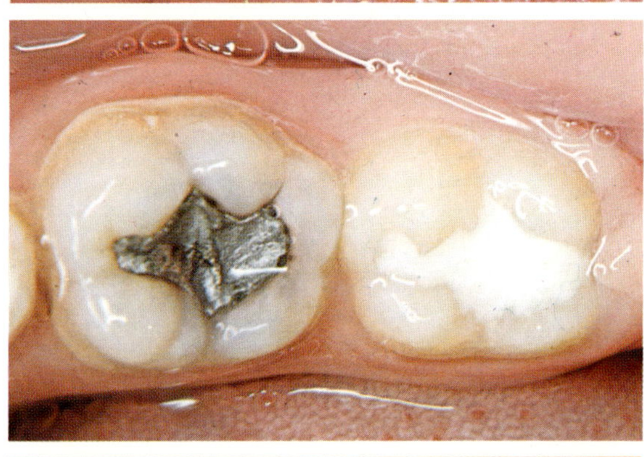

Fig. II-6 Patient K. B. Immediately after sealing with 3M Concise Brand White Sealant. The sealant will block out the caries-susceptible grooves forming a smooth margin with the enamel cuspal slopes. The adjacent first molar is highly exposed to secondary caries at the amalgam margins. The brighter of the two white colors seen in Fig. II-4 was chosen by 3M Company for their White Sealant.

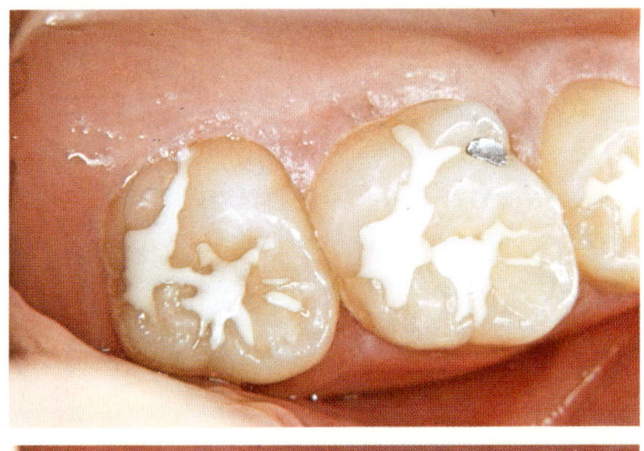

Fig. II-7 Patient N. S. The excellent retention of 3M White Sealant can be seen in this case 6 months after application. The sealant can be placed up to, or even over, old amalgam restorations. Note the lingual retention of the material.

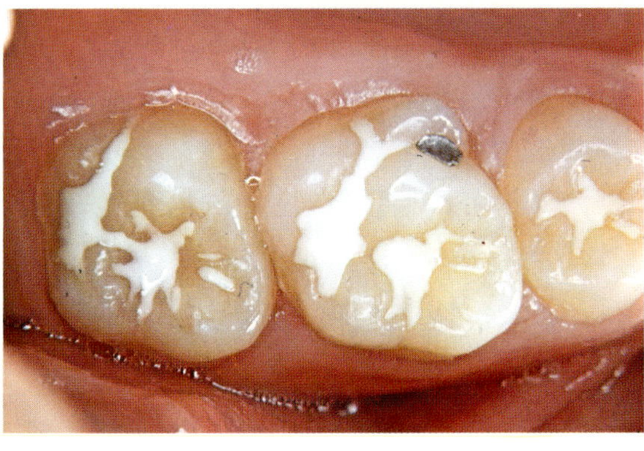

Fig. II-8 Patient N. S. The same case as seen in Fig. II-7 12 months after application. The only area of noticeable wear is on the oblique ridge of the first permanent molar. Excellent lingual retention is still apparent as is the retention of small areas within supplemental grooves.

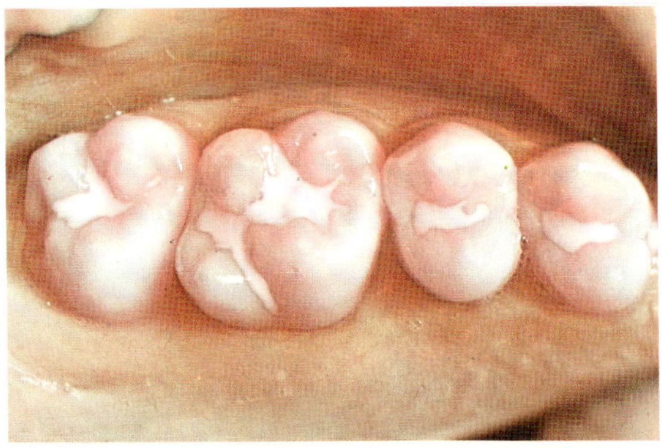

Fig. II-9   Patient S. E. A quadrant of bicuspids and permanent molars seen 6 months after application of 3M White Sealant.

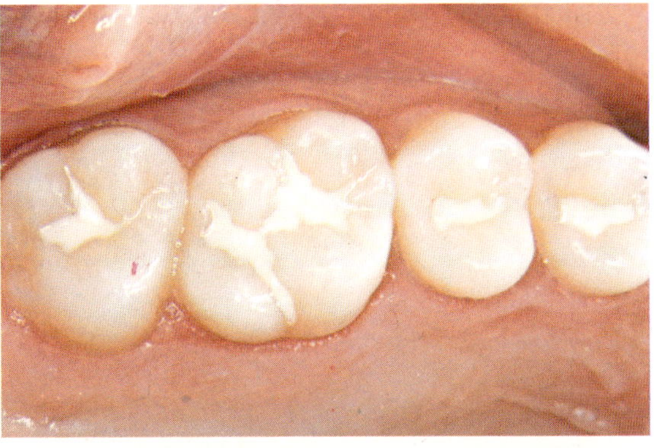

Fig. II-10   Patient S. E. The same quadrant as seen in Fig. II-9 12 months after sealant application. The only visible wear is on the oblique ridge area of the first molar.

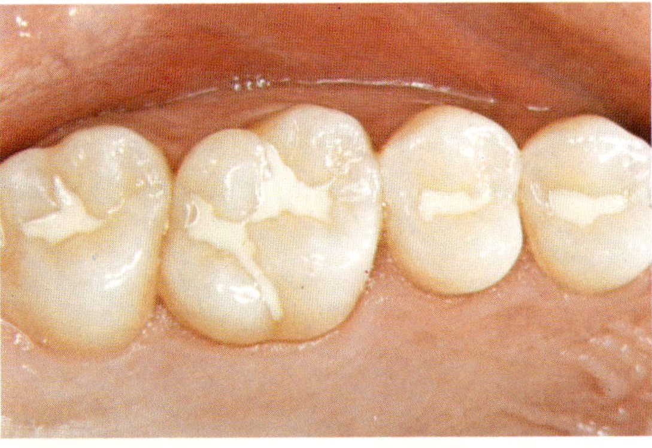

Fig. II-11   Patient S. E. After 18 months, the quadrant as seen in the previous figures shows no further appreciable wear or loss of sealant. Excellent retention such as this was the rule with the 3M White Sealant, and accurate assessment of retention is made possible by the coloring agent in the sealant.

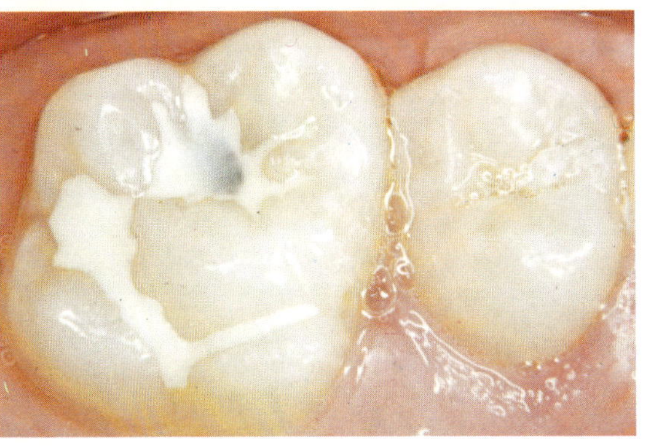

Fig. II-12   Patient D. S. The small occlusal amalgam seen under the sealant was covered 12 months previously during a routine sealant application appointment. Although the amalgam surface may soon again be exposed, due to wear of the sealant, the life of the amalgam will have been extended by eliminating marginal leakage. Note again excellent lingual retention of the material.

Fig. II-13   Patient K. I. There was no diagnosable caries around the small occlusal amalgam in the first permanent molar. The adjacent grooves are, however, extremely susceptible to secondary caries attack. In the course of a routine sealant treatment such amalgams can be covered with sealant. This tooth is seen after acid etching and exhibits the characteristic frosty-white appearance of etched enamel.

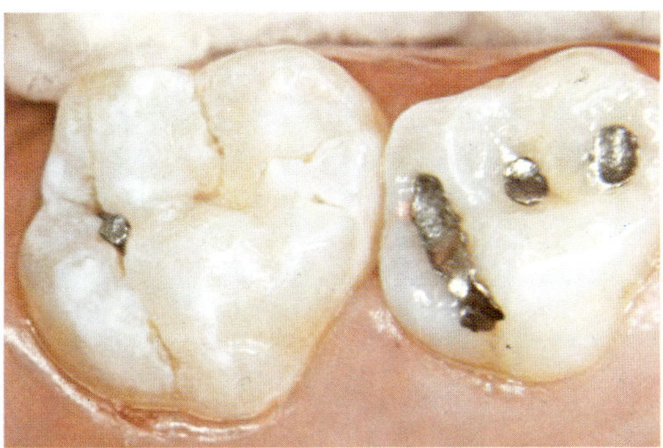

Fig. II-14   Patient K. I. 3M White Sealant was applied and the old amalgam restoration completely covered. This treatment is certainly more beneficial than leaving the situation as in Fig. II-13. It could be argued that the amalgam should be replaced with a more extensive amalgam, but this entails the irreversible removal of healthy tooth structure which can be avoided with diligent use of a sealant.

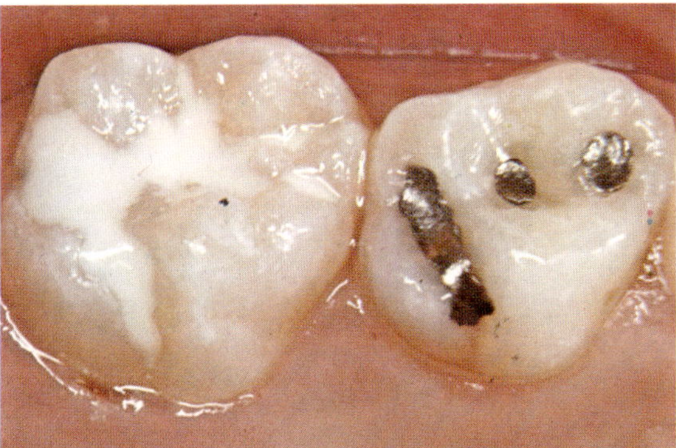

Fig. II-15   Patient C. A. This type of occlusal surface is frequently seen and is one that is obviously very susceptible to caries. Removal of all stain and fissure anatomy would result in a large occlusal amalgam which can be avoided with use of a sealant. The disto-marginal ridge is still covered with gingival tissue which will interfere with sealant application in this area.

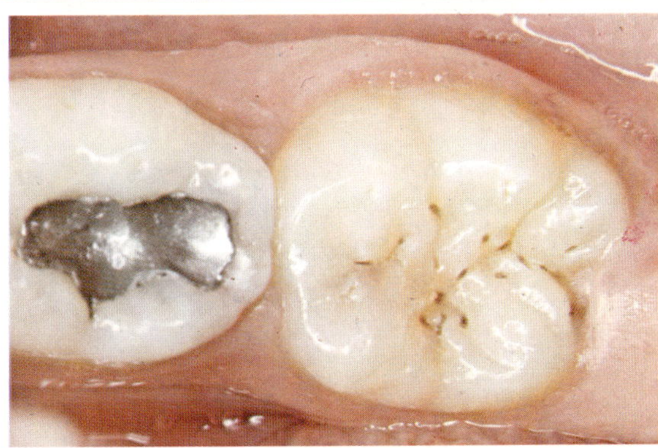

Fig. II-16   Patient C. A. Simple seating of a matrix band, such as this Caulk AutoMatrix, will retract the tissue and allow sealant application to the previously covered grooves. Gingival retraction cord can also sometimes be used to expose sub-gingival grooves. Rubber dam application is the ideal solution to most cases of gingival interference where a simpler solution is not satisfactory.

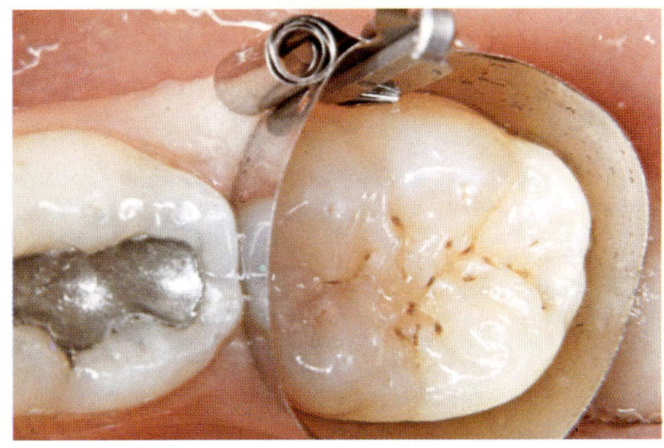

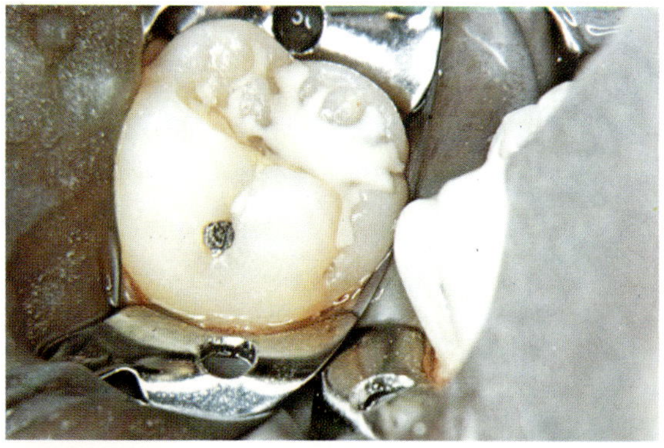

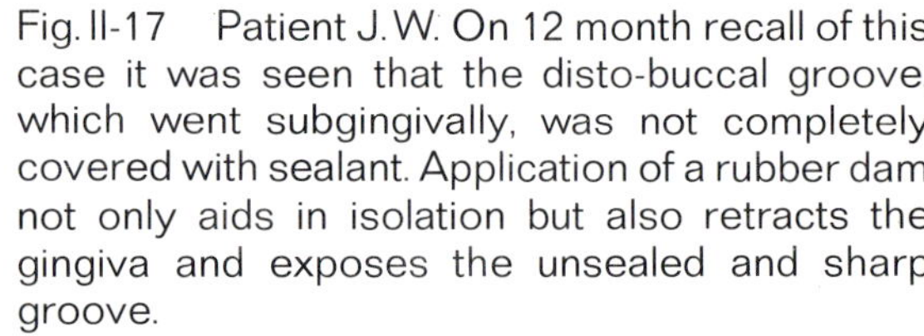

Fig. II-17   Patient J.W. On 12 month recall of this case it was seen that the disto-buccal groove, which went subgingivally, was not completely covered with sealant. Application of a rubber dam not only aids in isolation but also retracts the gingiva and exposes the unsealed and sharp groove.

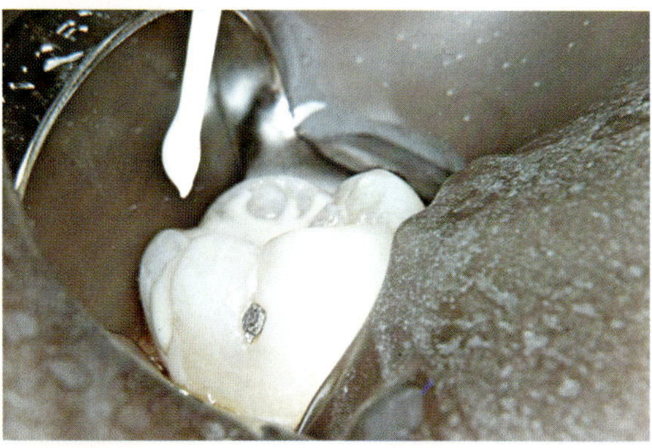

Fig. II-18   Patient J.W. Utilizing the sharp end of the 3M applicator brush, (Fig. II-32), sealant can be applied to small areas of troublesome accessibility. A similar tip is also found on the Caulk brush available with Nuva-Cote sealant (Fig. II-32).

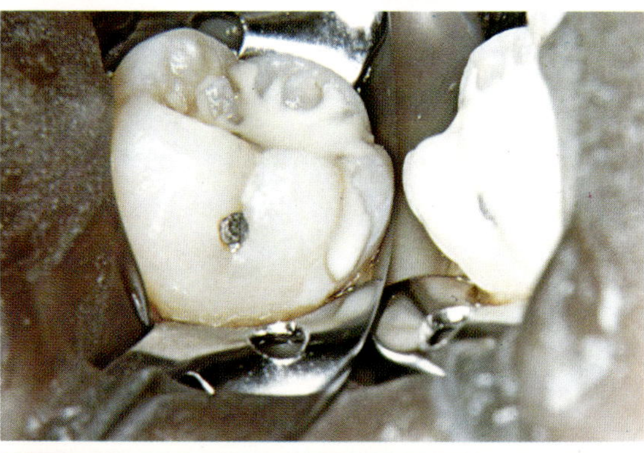

Fig. II-19   Patient J.W. Successful application of sealant to subgingival grooves assures caries-protection to otherwise exposed areas. Observe also the sealant retained in the buccal groove 12 months after application.

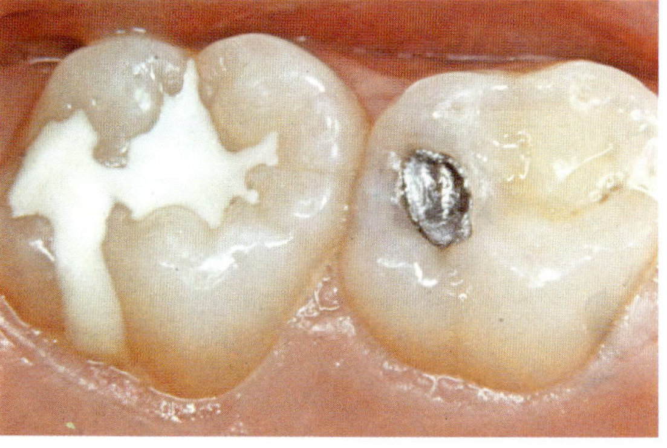

Fig. II-20   Patient C.E. This 12 month recall shows the retention of subgingival sealant application. In this case rubber dam was not used but the gingival sulcus was packed with gingival retraction cord prior to etching and sealing. The subgingival groove was successfully sealed without moisture contamination.

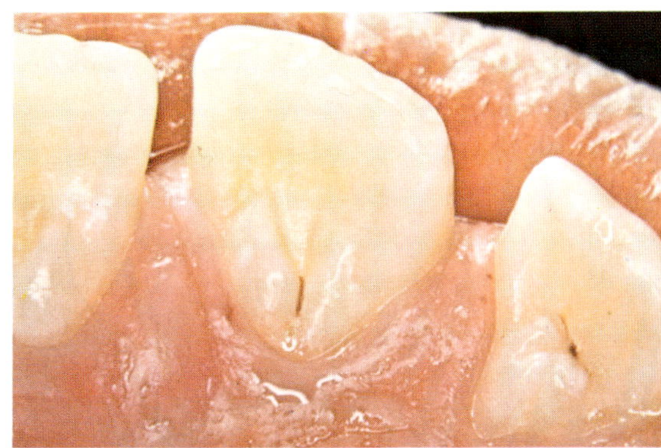

Fig. II-21   Patient J. F. Lingual pits on the anterior teeth are also ideal for sealant application. Careful examination for caries must be undertaken prior to sealing, particularly on lateral incisors where x-rays should be checked for invaginations.

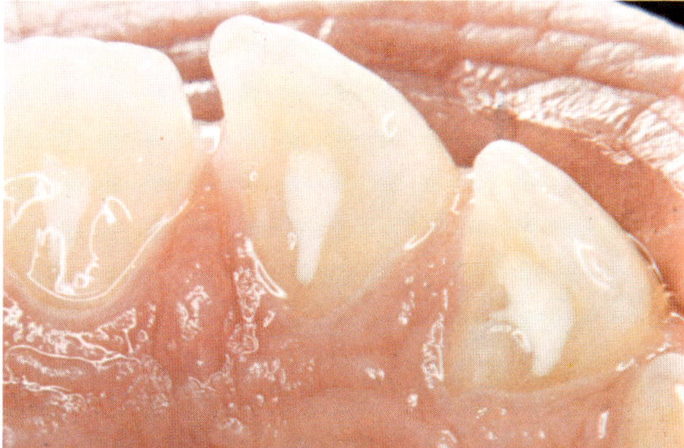
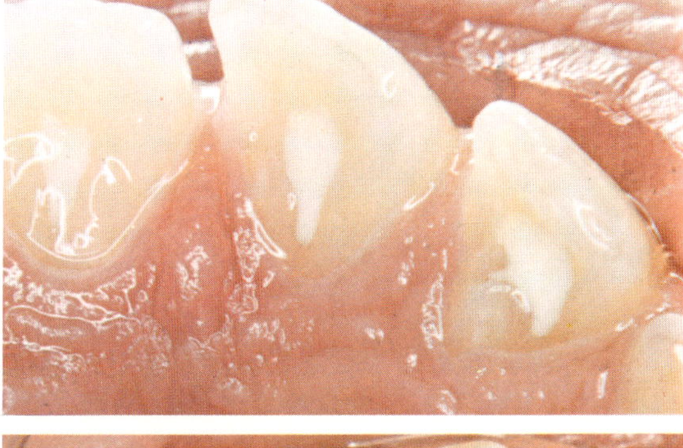

Fig. II-22   Patient J. F. 6 month recall photograph of the previous case sealed with 3M White Sealant.

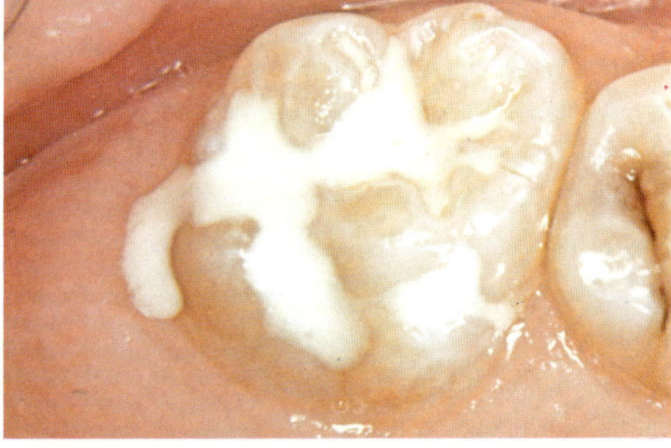

Fig. II-23   Patient T. S. Frequently with partially erupted first permanent molars where grooves are close to gingival tissue, the sealant will flow onto the adjacent gingiva. Rather than trying to wipe off the material before polymerization, or flick it off after polymerization, it is best to trim the excess material down after polymerization with a fluted composite finishing bur (Fig. V-5).

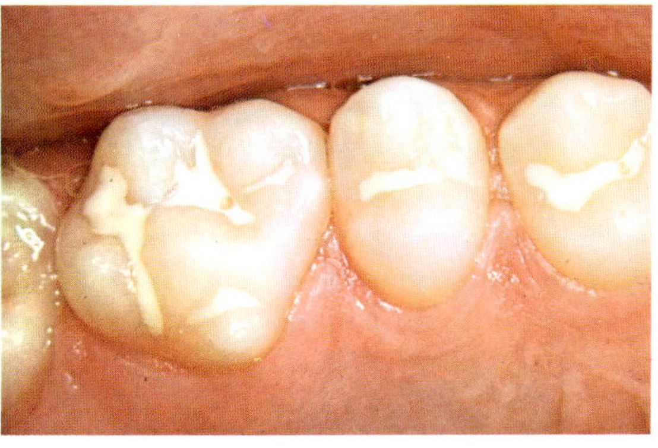

Fig. II-24   Patient K. H. Bubbles can frequently form when mixing resin sealants. They pose no particular problem as long as they do not penetrate to the depth of the fissure or, by location, weaken the sealant. Careful mixing and application can eliminate most bubbles. Seen here is a 12 month recall photograph showing a bubble present since application.

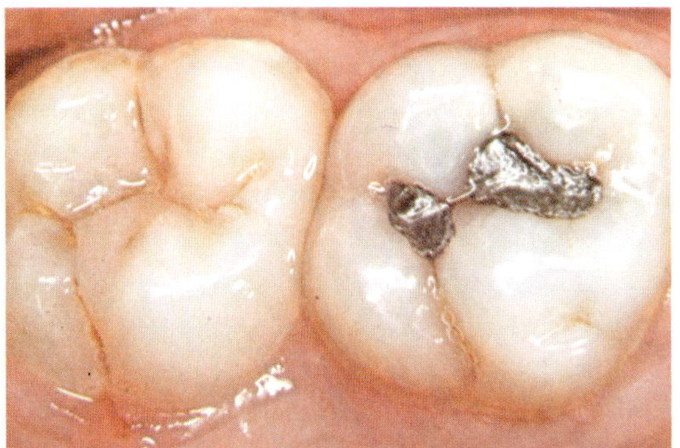

Fig. II-25   Patient M. M. As seen in Figs. II-12 to 14, amalgam can be successfully covered with sealant to reduce marginal leakage, extend the life of the amalgam and protect adjacent caries-susceptible grooves. As the amalgam increases in size the sealant retentive area is decreased. Thus it would not be recommended to seal over amalgams larger than seen in this first molar.

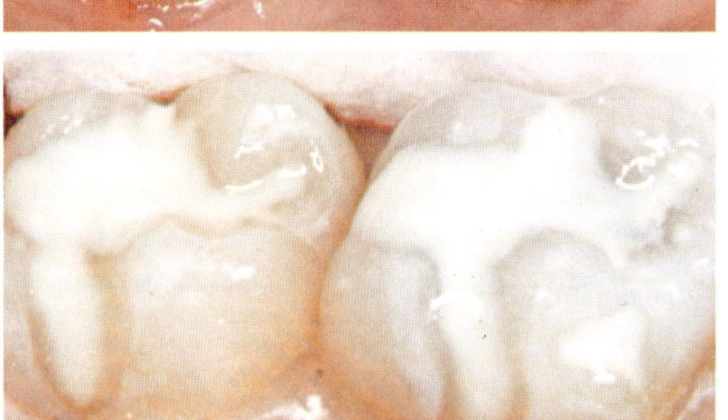

Fig. II-26   Patient M. M. Immediately after application of sealant to Fig. II-25. Sealant should be applied approximately half-way up the cuspal slopes. Note that the etched area of enamel is still visible beyond the sealant margin. This ensures that no sealant is covering unetched enamel which would result in "lifting" of the margin.

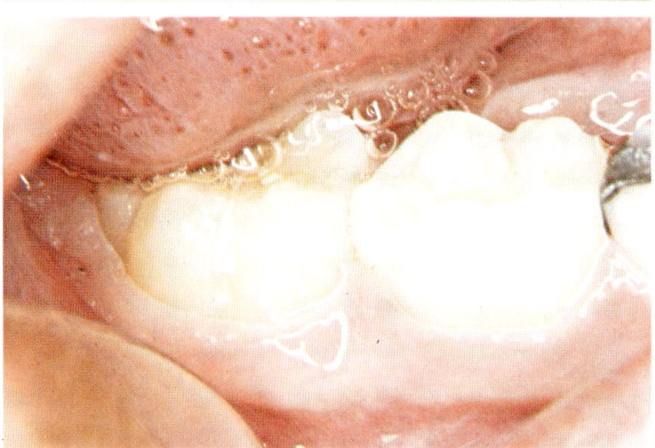

Fig. II-27   Patient N. K. The only sealant loss seen at 6 and 12 months was on the buccal of lower permanent molars or the lingual of upper permanent molars. This patient (15 month recall photograph) exhibits a large tongue and profusive salivary flow, which makes isolation without rubber dam very difficult. Salivary contamination of etched enamel will result in sealant loss as seen in this case of partial sealant loss from the buccal groove.

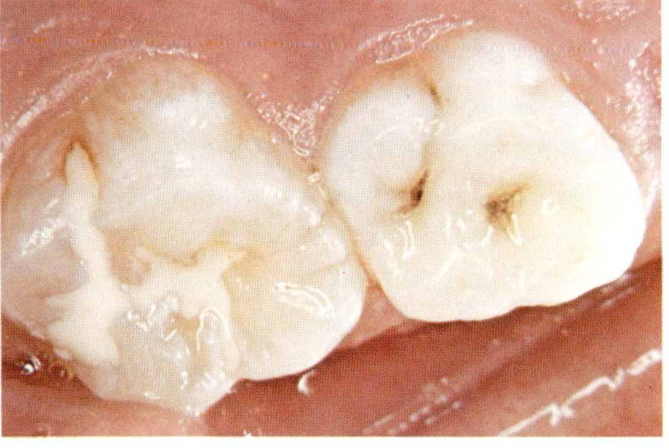

Fig. II-28   Patient J. H. At the 12 month recall a brown stain was seen at the base of the lingual groove. Explorer examination revealed that the margin of sealant in this area was slightly "lifted" from the enamel surface enabling the oral fluid to circulate under this area of sealant.

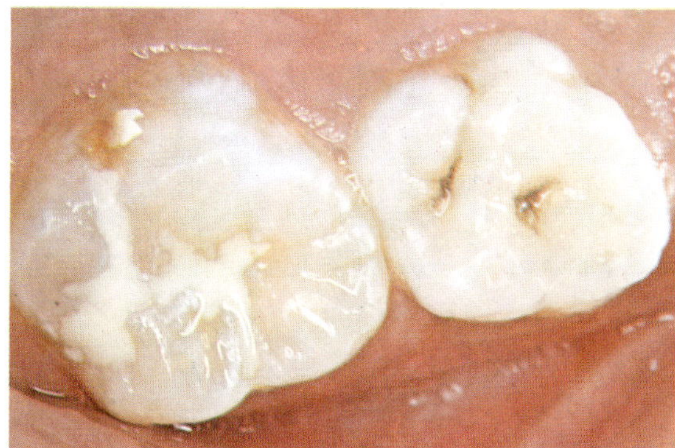

Fig. II-29   Patient J.H. After lifting up and breaking off the unattached sealant the area was thoroughly cleaned and re-etched. It is thought that the poor sealant bonding was a result either of insufficient plaque removal in the lingual groove, or contamination of the etched groove by crevicular fluids from the adjacent gingival margin prior to sealant placement.

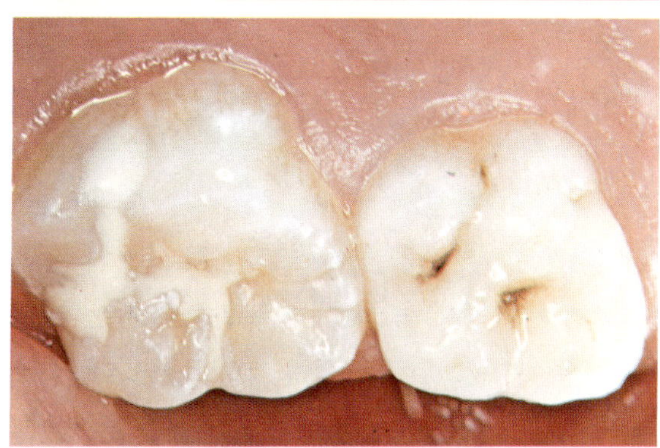

Fig. II-30   Patient J.H. The lingual groove after re-sealing. If plaque is properly removed from such grooves, isolation is maintained and the etched area of enamel is adequate for sealant placement, there is no reason to see any leakage or "lifting" of sealant margins. This is the only case of sealant leakage seen in over 2700 teeth studied.

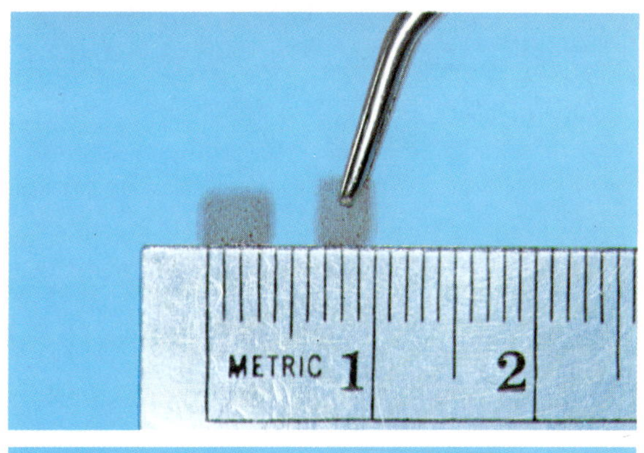

Fig. II-31   These small sponges are supplied with the 3M White Sealant. When held in a lockable cotton pliers the sponges are excellent for acid application during etching. For resin application the sponges are inadequate and their use is contraindicated.

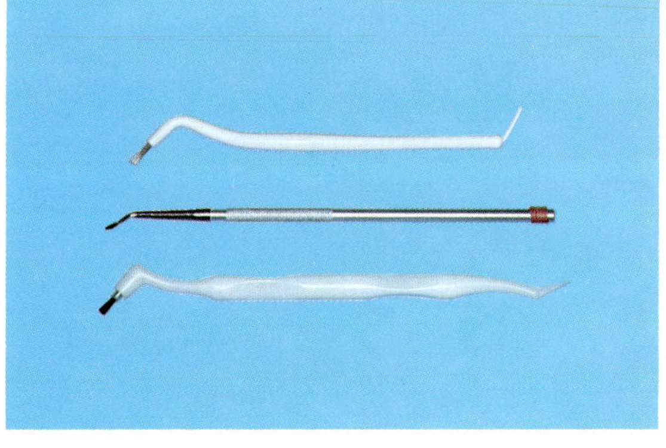

Fig. II-32   Three types of brushes suitable for sealant application. Top: disposable brush available from the 3M Company, St. Paul, Minnesota. Middle: a sable hair brush distributed with AlphaSeal, Amalgamated Dental, London. Bottom: a brush with a disposable tip as supplied with Nuva-Cote, L. D. Caulk Company, Milford, Delaware. Disposable brushes are desirable with auto-polymerizing resin systems.

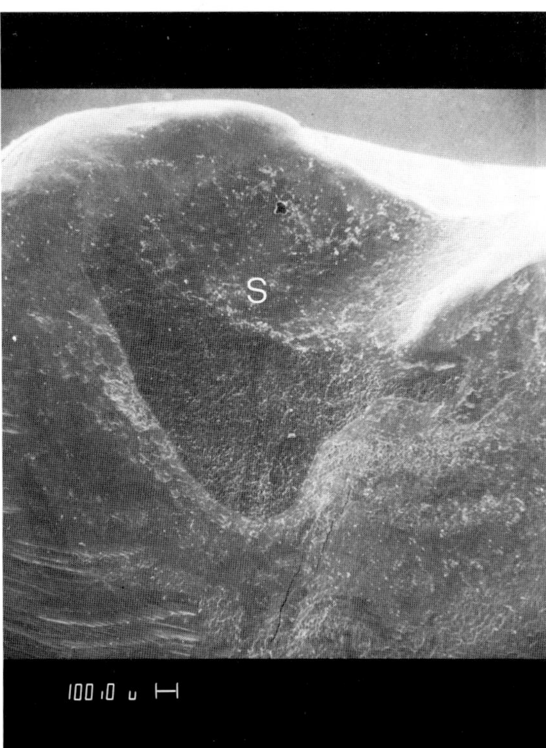

Fig. II-33   Patient W. G. A scanning electron photomicrograph of a bicuspid that was extracted for orthodontic reasons 18 months after sealant (AlphaSeal) application. A section was cut through the tooth bucco-lingually to show sealant (S) adaptation to the occlusal fissure. No evidence of a break in the sealant/enamel bond can be seen.

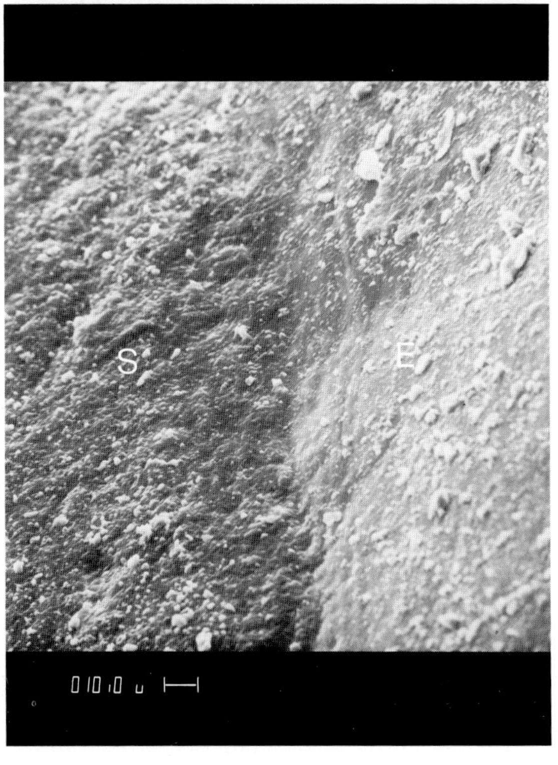

Fig. II-34   Patient W. G. A higher power view of the sealant (S)–enamel (E) interface. There is no sign of any marginal breakdown or "lifting" of the sealant at the margin, even after 18 months. This, and other examples examined under SEM, support the contention that sealants applied according to the proper technique will not leak from "lifting" of margins as some operators fear.

Fig. II-35   Patient K. P. The future of sealants? Perhaps interproximal sealing is not so far away. There is certainly a vast potential for caries protection of interproximal surfaces–possibly with a fluoride-containing sealant, or a temporary sealant over a fluoride-treated etch of enamel. The challenge is there!

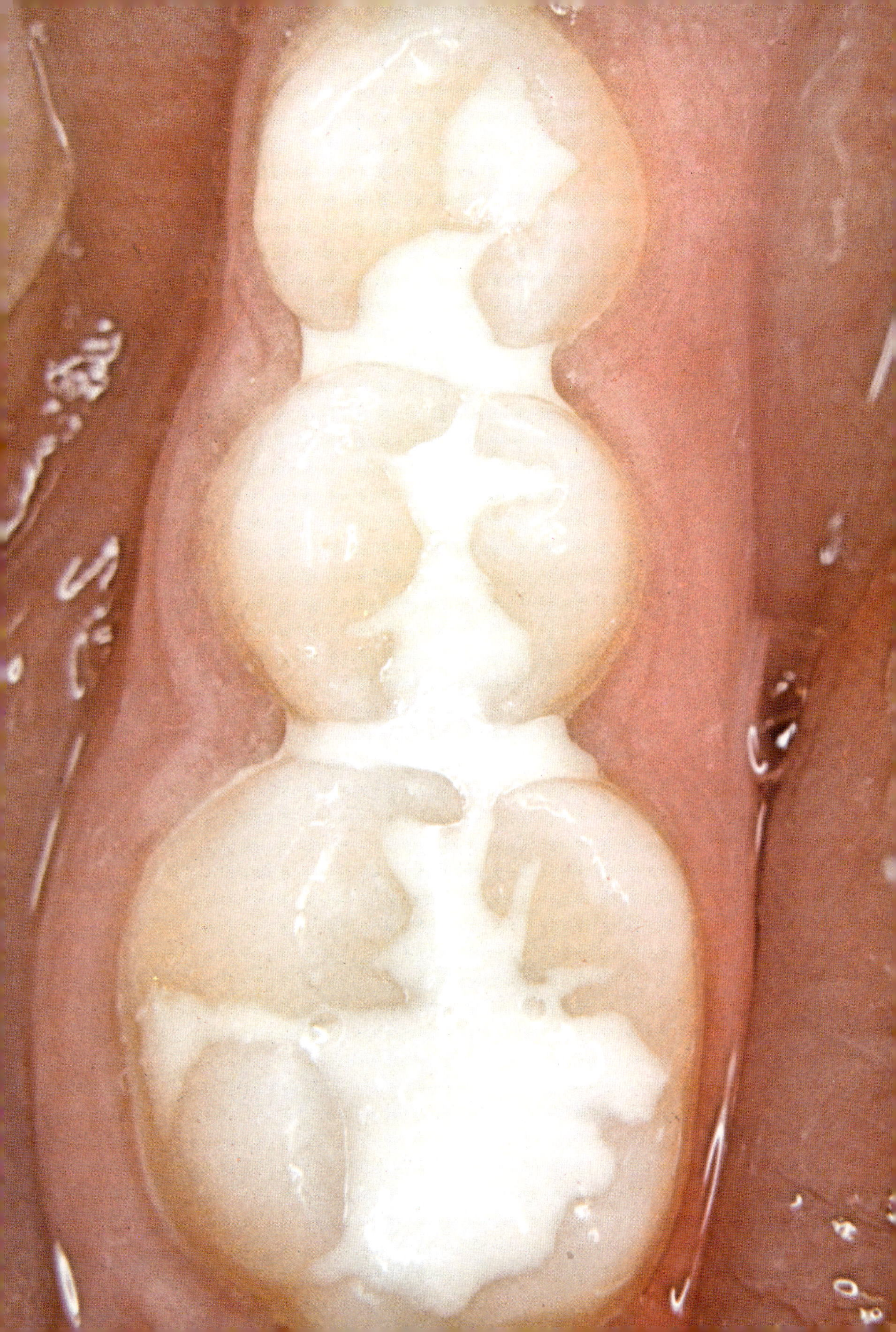

References

1. *Ast, D. B., Smith, D. J., Wachs, B., and Cantwell, K. T.:*
Newburgh-Kingston Caries-Fluorine Study XIV. Combined clinical and roentgenographic dental findings after ten years of fluoride experience. JADA 52: 314–325, 1956.

2. *Bodecker, C. F.:*
Enamel fissure eradication. NYSDJ 30: April 64, 149–154.

3. *Bodecker, C. F.:*
Dental caries immunization without filling. NYSDJ 30: October 6, 337.

4. *Buonocore, M. G.:*
The Use of Adhesives in Dentistry. Charles C. Thomas, Publisher, Springfield, Illinois, 1975.

5. *Charbeneau, G. T., Dennison, J. B., and Ryge, G.:*
A filled pit and fissure sealant: 18-month results. JADA, 95: 299–306, 1977.

6. *Chow, L. C. and Brown, W. E.:*
Topical fluoridation of teeth before sealant application. J. Dent. Res. 54: 1089, 1975.

7. *Cons, N. C., Pollard, S. T. and Leske, G. S.:*
Adhesive Sealant Clinical Trial: results of a three-year study in a fluoridated area. J. Prev. Dent. 3: 14–19, 1976.

8. *Gwinnett, A. J.:*
The bonding of sealants to enamel. J. Am. Soc. Prev. Dent. 1: 21–29, 1973.

9. *Gwinnett, A. J., Buonocore, M. G., and Sheykholeslam, Z.:*
Effect of fluoride on etched human and bovine tooth enamel surfaces as demonstrated by scanning electron microscopy. Arch. Oral Biol. 17: 271–278, 1972.

10. *Handelman, S. L., Washburn, F., and Wopperer, P.:*
Two-year report of sealant effect on bacteria in dental caries. JADA, 93: 967–970, 1976.

11. *Horowitz, H. S., Heifetz, S. B., and Poulsen, S.:*
Retention and effectiveness of an adhesive sealant after five years. AADR abstract no. 72, J. Dent. Res., June 1977.

12. *Hyatt, T. P.:*
Prophylactic odontotomy. Dent. Cosmos, March 1923.

13. *Ibsen, R. L. and Neville, K.:*
Adhesive Restorative Dentistry. W. B. Saunders Co., Philadelphia, 1974.

14. *Low, T., von Fraunhofer, J. A., and Winter, G. B.:*
Influence of the topical application of fluoride on the in vitro adhesion of fissure sealants. J. Dent. Res. 56: 17–20, 1977.

15. *Rock, W. P.:*
The effect of etching of human enamel upon bond strengths with fissure sealant resins. Arch. Oral Biol. 19: 873–877, 1974.

16. *Schachtele, Charles:*
Personal Communication

17. *Silverstone, L. M. and Dogon, I. L. (Eds.):*
Proceedings of an International Symposium on the Acid Etch Technique, p. 82, North Central Publishing Co., St. Paul, Minnesota, 1975.

18. *Silverstone, L. M.:*
Fissure sealants: The susceptibility to dissolution of acid-etched and subsequently abraded enamel. Caries Res. 11: 46–51, 1977.

19. *Silverstone, L. M.:*
Personal Communication.

20. *Simonsen, R. J. and Stallard, R. E.:*
Fissure sealants: Colored sealant retention 3 months post application. Quintessence Int. 8: 1–6, 1977.

21. *Simonsen, R. J.:*
Clinical retention of 3M White Sealant with 5% Sodium Fluoride addition. Unpublished.

22. *Stiles, H. M., Ward, G. T., Woolridge, E. D., and Meyers, R.:*
Adhesive sealant clinical trial: Comparative results of application by a dentist or dental auxiliaries. J. Prev. Dent. 3: 8–11, 1976.

23. *Swartz, M. L. et al.:*
Addition of fluoride to pit and fissure sealants—a feasibility study. J. Dent. Res. 55: 757–771, 1976.

Chapter 3

Anterior Fracture Restoration and Finishing of Composites

Probably none of the uses of the acid etch technique described here, are as challenging, rewarding and frequently needed, as the restoration of fractured incisors. Facial trauma from automobile and bicycle accidents, sporting injuries (particularly in northern climates from ice hockey and ice skating) and pugilism, can frequently lead to fractures of the anterior teeth.

The days when child accident victims were further traumatized, (psychologically), by having to go through many years of childhood and adolescence with fractured central incisors, (Fig. III-1), or worse yet, with stainless steel crowns covering the fracture sites, (Fig. III-13), are thankfully gone forever. There is, now, no excuse for delaying restoration, or temporarily placing stainless steel crowns until such a time as pulpal conditions permit the placement of full crowns. This was the accepted, and only, treatment some years ago. The development, however, of dental composite resins and the acid etch technique, has opened up a simple, rapid, inexpensive and highly esthetic restorative procedure for the treatment of fractured incisors. The composite restoration of fractured incisors has been considered a temporary procedure. The technique has now developed to a stage where it should be considered, as any other restoration, semi-permanent requiring occasional ongoing observation and possible touch-up.

Technique

Two basic techniques of anterior fracture restoration are common, irrespective of whether the ultraviolet curing or autopolymerizing resin systems are used.

The first, as detailed by *Buonocore*,[2] involves no tooth preparation, and an overlapping of the composite resin onto labial and lingual enamel. This overlap involves etching a considerable amount of the labial and lingual enamel and feather-edging a veneer of composite onto these surfaces.

The second, as explained by this author,[10] involves bevelling the enamel margin around the fracture line and finishing the composite to the margin finish line produced. This technique is very similar to the chamfer technique advocated by *Jordan* et al.[6]

There are no advantages of the feather-edge technique over the bevel technique. The only possible advantage would be one of greater retention since a much larger area of enamel is used for bonding. That advantage, however, becomes academic, when one considers that bevelled restorations do not have a tendency to be lost due to insufficient retention. The bevelled preparation to be described here, provides more than adequate retention based on three years of using the technique by this author (one example is seen in Figures III-18 to 20) and by *Jordan* et al., (97.1% retention).

Disadvantages of feather-edged restorations are several. The application of a composite layer on top of labial and lingual enamel invariably results in over-contouring the tooth. This, in turn, may result in occlusal interferences, as well as an esthetically less desirable restoration. In addition, the feather-edging of the composite makes for a weak area in the restoration where the composite is thinnest, leading to marginal breakdown and marginal staining (Fig. III-7).

The only disadvantages to the bevel restoration are that tooth structure must be removed, and that it is sometimes more difficult to match the color of the restoration to the tooth, since the transition from composite to enamel is more abrupt with the bevel type preparation, than with the feather-edge. The removal of tooth structure is, however, very minimal and is only in an area where the enamel prisms are longitudinally exposed already. Color match is similarly, rarely a problem.

Enamel prisms are oriented at 90° to the enamel surface. These prisms, when traumatically fractured, separate along their longitudinal axes. By placing a bevel along the fractured margin all the way around the tooth, the enamel prisms, on the slope of the bevel, are "end-on", and in the ideal orientation for creation of the desired etching pattern. The bevel, Figure III-2, is placed with a pointed or round-nosed (*Jordan*) diamond, or even a 7901 FG fluted composite finishing bur in the high-speed handpiece. The bevel should be about 1–1.5 mm wide and should be at about 45° to the surface. This preparation not only provides all the freshly prepared enamel necessary for bonding, but it also leaves a definite finishing line to which the composite is finished.

All exposed dentin should be protected with a calcium hydroxide base, (Procal or Dycal are excellent—Procal seems to be less soluble in phosphoric acid and is recommended for use when acid etching is necessary). Figure III-3 shows a lingual view of the based fractures. Care should be taken not to leave any base on the enamel bevel. If there is a question of enough retention, either because of the size of the fracture or because of the occlusion, the bevel can be widened. The enamel bevel is then etched for 60 seconds with, (in this case), 37% phosphoric acid. Any composite system can be similarly used, but the case seen here used the 3M Concise Enamel Bond System. When etching is complete and the enamel has been thoroughly washed for at least 30 seconds with an air/water spray, (Ref. Chapter II–p. 21), the Enamel Bond unfilled resin can be applied, (with a disposable brush), to the frosty-white appearing etched enamel. The Concise filled resin is then immediately added, either in a previously adapted crown form, or simply with a Mylar strip matrix.

Finishing

Gross contouring of the excess composite can be done with high-speed diamond burs after polymerization. Fine contouring should be done with two composite fluted finishing burs, both from Midwest American. For labial and interproximal finishing, the 7901 FG is best, (Fig. V-5), while the 7408 FG (Fig. VII-5) is excellent for lingual finishing to the bevelled line. Using the finishing burs dry, will enable the operator to clearly see when the margin is reached.

Discs are used as the final step in finishing, unless glazing is contemplated, in which case it is not necessary to use discs prior to glazing. Figure III-4 shows one of the best discs available for finishing composites, the 3M Sof-Lex Brand Finishing and Polishing Discs. These discs give composites a remarkably smooth surface that is far smoother than that obtained by any previous disc. These discs are very pliable, and care must be taken not to put too much pressure on them, or the brass center ring may contact the restoration.

Glazing of composites is recommended, and

the last part of this chapter will deal with some clinical research results into glazing. Any of the commercially available unfilled resins can be used as a glaze layer, although care must be taken to apply a thick enough layer for polymerization. A thin layer will not polymerize due to the inhibiting effect of the oxygen in the atmosphere.

In Figure III-5 a glaze layer, (3M experimental glaze), has been applied to the right central and to half of the left central. Prior to applying the glaze, a re-etch (or double etch) of the marginal enamel is recommended. About 2 mm of enamel all the way around the composite margin is etched and washed. The glaze is then applied to the composite, (to which it will chemically bond), over the margin of the restoration and onto the area of etched enamel, to which the glaze will mechanically bond. This, in effect, completely seals off the restoration from marginal breakdown and is insurance against any marginal leakage. The technique has been performed in this manner for over three years by the author with gratifying results (Fig. III-18 to 29).

The left central incisor (Fig. III-5) was only half glazed, as it was part of a study to examine the surface wear of the Sof-Lex disc finish, (mesial portion of the restoration), compared to a glaze finish. When the glaze is newly applied and the rest of the tooth is dry, the glaze is clearly visible. However, after washing, (Fig. II-6), the glaze layer blends in very well with tooth enamel (also Fig. III-8).

The necessity of an intermediate unfilled resin layer between etched enamel and the filled composite is the subject of some controversy in the literature. *Dreyer Jorgensen*,[4] *Raadal*,[8] *Asmussen*[1] and *Ulvestad*[11] form a Scandinavian block that seems to believe that the intermediate layer is superfluous. They believe that there is sufficient unfilled resin available in a filled resin for adequate "tag" penetration. There seems, on the other hand, plentiful evidence that the intermediate resin layer decreases micro-leakage.[3,5] Since apparently no researcher is claiming any harmful effects from an intermediate resin layer, no reason can be seen to omit the step, as the amount of time it takes to put on is insignificant.

Some of the disadvantages of the feather-edge type preparation, (marginal breakdown and marginal staining of the feather-edge), are seen in Figure III-7. The actual fracture was much smaller than the bulky labial composite layer would indicate. After removal of the old restoration, a new restoration was placed using the bevel technique, 3M Enamel Bond and Cosmic (Amalgamated Dental, London), Figure III-8. Cosmic has a slightly lighter color tone than Concise's universal shade, and was thus chosen for this case.

Mandibular incisors and a maxillary lateral restored with Concise and glazed, are seen in Figures III-9 to 12.

Some of the problems with stainless steel crowns, (poor esthetics, poor adaptation, gingival irritation, secondary caries), are shown in Figures III-13 and 14. Restoration of these fractures is sometimes complicated by the preparation made in order to accommodate the crown (Fig. III-15). When fractures extend subgingivally (as they frequently do on the lingual), a special effort must be made to place a smooth composite. Electrosurgery or a localized gingivectomy may be necessary to adequately expose the fracture margin.

Glaze finish

The benefits of a glaze surface have been documented previously.[9]

Critics of glazing contend that the soft unfilled resin will rapidly wear away. Some in vitro studies, of questionable validity for the in vivo situation, show rapid wear of glaze as a toothbrushing machine is let loose on the resin stubs. Initial problems with glazing, were not with rapid wear, but with non-polymerization. An unfilled resin must be applied in a thick layer for polymerization to occur. If this is not done, areas of the glaze will not polymerize as the oxygen in the atmosphere inhibits the reaction. This will leave islands of glaze and areas of exposed filled resin. The operator may not be aware that the glaze has not polymerized, and on recall, when the glaze is not present, he may incorrectly conclude that the glaze has worn away. Figures III-19 and 20 show 1 and 3-year recall photographs of an incisal fracture, (pre-op. Fig. III-18), which was restored using the Nuva System. The ultraviolet system technique is basically the same as the autopolymerizing technique, except that the Nuva-Fil composite must be added in small amounts to ensure polymerization by the ultraviolet light, which can only penetrate, (and therefore polymerize), to a depth of approximately 1.5 mm. Nuva-Seal was used as a glaze layer after the enamel margins of the restoration were re-etched.

Figure III-19, the one-year recall photograph, shows clinically the presence of the glaze layer. The fracture restoration can be detected by comparing Figures III-19 to the pre-restoration photograph, Figure III-18. Looking closely at the light reflection on the mesial portion of the tooth, sharp light reflection can be seen from the enamel. As this reflective area is followed down towards the composite, the light reflection is interrupted by a wedge-shaped area of un-glazed composite. Further down, the light reflection is once again detectable as a dull sheen as it reflects from the glaze layer present. Close inspection of the photograph will reveal the visible glaze layer covering the composite/ enamel margin, (after the re-etch), as is more clearly seen on the SEM photographs. The light reflection on the 3-year recall (Fig. III-20) is not quite so clear for showing the glaze layer, but the wedge-shaped composite layer, seen on the SEM photographs, can still be observed.

A negative replica was taken at each yearly recall. One side of an acetate replicating tape, (Ladd Industries, Burlington, Vermont), was softened with acetone, applied to the labial surface with moderate pressure and allowed to harden before careful removal. Under the scanning electron microscope, these replicas reveal evidence of Nuva-Seal present as a glaze layer at 1, 2 and 3-year recall appointments, with very little wear being evident, Figures III-21 to 29. The wedge-shaped area that is not glazed, was more than likely a good example of a too-thin layer of glaze being applied, and hence polymerization did not occur. It is interesting to compare the 1, 2 and 3-year photographs under increasing power to observe the composite filler particles becoming more exposed with time as the softer composite matrix wears down.

This series of photomicrographs shows conclusively that even unfilled resins not specifically designed for glazing, will function well as an outer layer on composite restorations for up to three years. It also shows that non-glazed composite becomes slightly rougher with time, as the matrix is worn faster than the filler particles. The photomicrographs illustrate the excellent marginal integrity of a bevelled anterior fracture restoration after three years, and demonstrate that re-etching the enamel margin prior to glazing can result in the margin being completely sealed for three years.

Improvement in glaze materials should make re-etching, and the subsequent addition of a glaze of resin, the method of choice in finishing composite restorations. There will always be a need for discs and strips for polishing composite restorations, for access limits the use of a glaze. However, in anterior fracture restoration, where access is no problem, glazing is recommended.

The perfection of the glaze technique in conjunction with a re-etch of enamel margins, and use of the bevel preparation, will eliminate the major problems encountered with anterior fracture restorations—namely, marginal breakdown and marginal staining.

There is no doubt, from the results of more than 3 years clinical study of glazes, that:

1. Glazes, when properly applied, will remain as a smooth overlay to composite restorations, providing the glaze polymerizes as a complete layer upon application.
2. A glaze layer can be effectively used to completely seal the margins of composite restorations.
3. Non-glazed filled resin becomes slightly rougher with time as more filler particles are exposed.
4. A glaze layer will give a smoother surface to a composite restoration by far, (and secondarily, a better color match over time as less stain is picked up), than any polishing technique available prior to the 3M Sof-Lex disc, up to 3 years after application.
5. The initial impression comparing glaze to Sof-Lex discs is that the glaze is somewhat smoother at times up to 12 months after application.

Study of an experimental glaze will be discussed in Chapter 5.

The author is indebted to Mr. *Jerry Mlinar* of 3M Company, who formulated the 5% submicron filled glaze used in all cases depicted in Chapters 3 and 5, except Figures III-18 to 29.

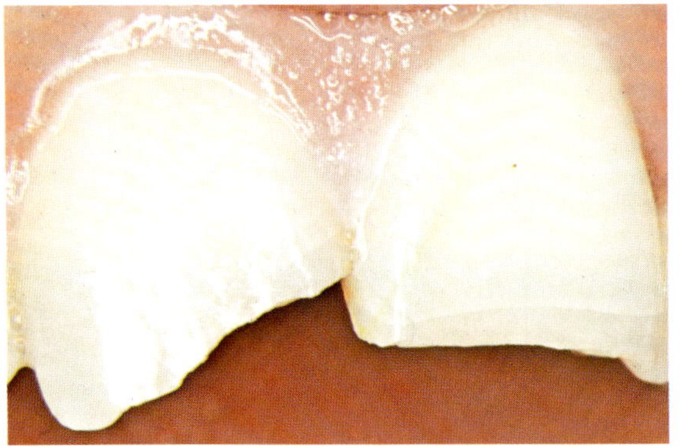

Fig. III-1   Patient J. H. A typical result of facial trauma, with both central incisors showing fractures into the dentin. It is unusual for other sequelae of trauma, such as mobility, subluxation or root fracture to be associated with crown fracture. The force of the blow is, in most cases, totally absorbed by the crown fracturing.

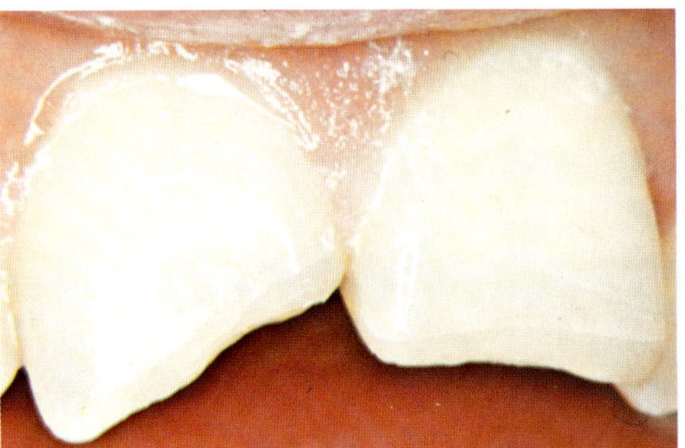

Fig. III-2   Patient J.H. The bevel preparation gives a line to which the composite can be finished. The result is a strong layer of composite bonded to a bevel about 1.5 mm wide at 45° to the enamel surface. The bevel removes all the longitudinally fractured enamel prisms and leaves enamel prisms in the bonding area in an "end-on" relation to the surface, ideal for etching.

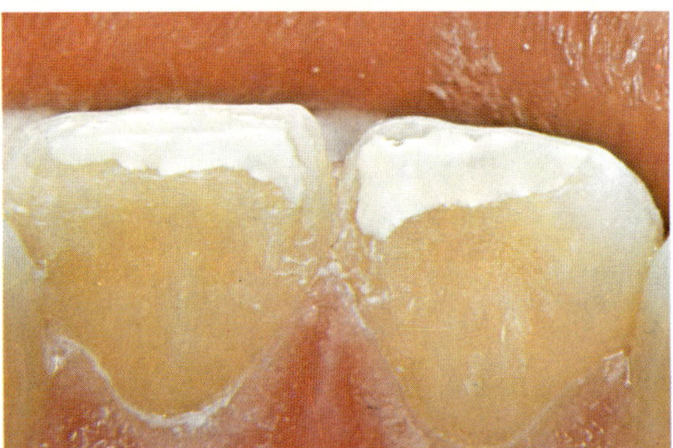

Fig. III-3   Patient J.H. All areas of exposed dentin should be covered with a calcium hydroxide base such as Procal or Dycal. Care should be taken to avoid excess base on enamel margins. The lingual bevel is made about the same size as the labial bevel, however if the size of the fracture requires an increase in retentive enamel area, the bevels can be increased in width.

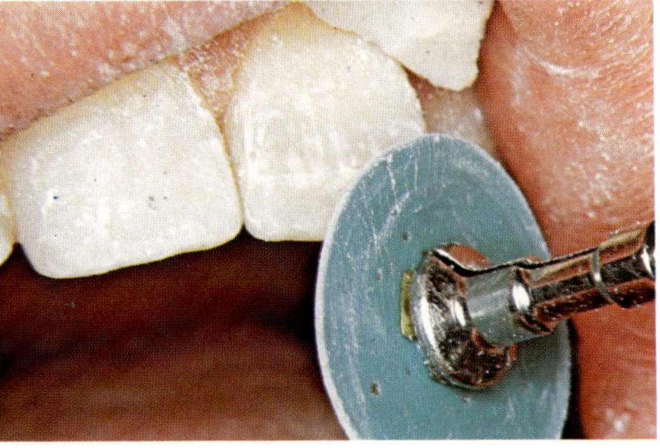

Fig. III-4   Patient J.H. After addition of 3M Enamel Bond and Concise using a Mylar strip as a matrix, the gross removal of excess composite can be accomplished using composite finishing burs. The best discs presently available (smoothest finish) are 3M Sof-Lex discs. These discs provide a finish almost as smooth as the addition of a glaze layer of unfilled resin.

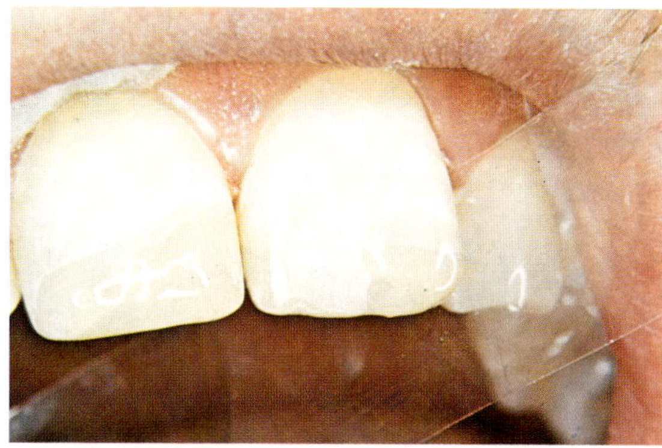

Fig. III-5　Patient J. H. The finishing of this case was completed with an experimental glaze layer on top of the Sof-Lex disc finish. The upper left central incisor was left with the mesial-half disced, and the distal-half glazed, to test the wear of the finishing techniques (Figs. V-21 and 22). Prior to glazing, the marginal enamel is etched again (about 2 mm wide) so that the glaze can seal the margin.

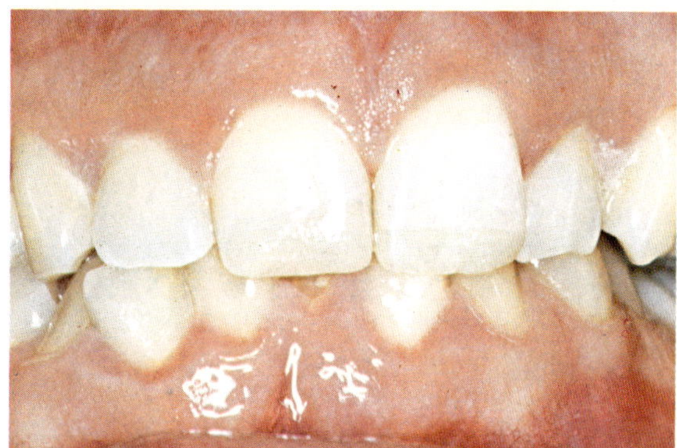

Fig. III-6　Patient J. H. The completed case in full mouth view.

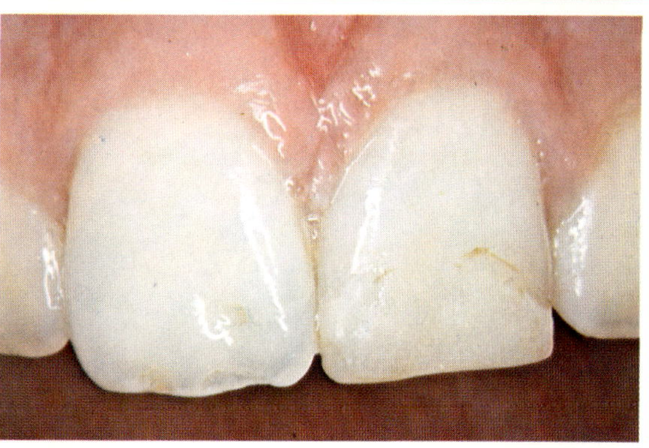

Fig. III-7　Patient T. J. This feather-edge anterior fracture restoration exhibits some of the disadvantages of feather-edge finishing—namely marginal breakdown and marginal staining. How long this restoration had been in place was not known, nor was known which material had been used. The old material was removed and the fracture restoration was redone.

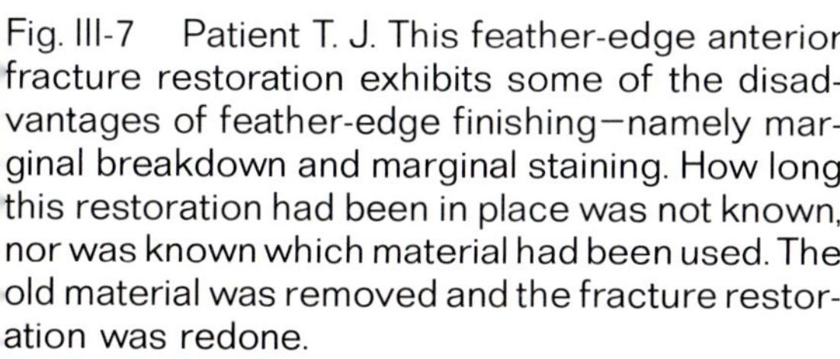

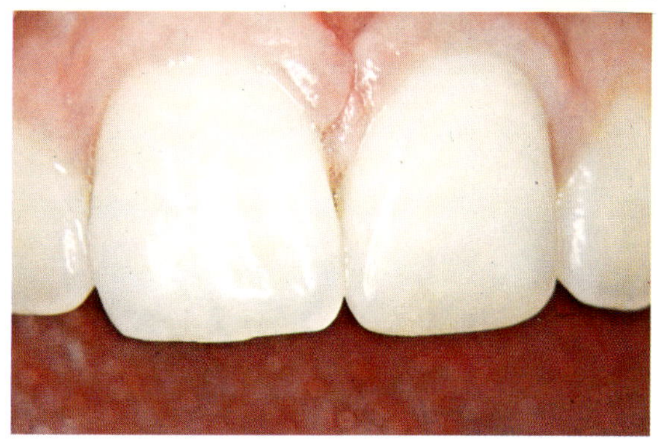

Fig. III-8　Patient T. J. After completion of the new restoration utilizing the bevel technique for preparation of the fractured margin. Much less of the labial enamel is now covered with composite and the bevelled finishing line will stand up to wear far better than the feather edge.

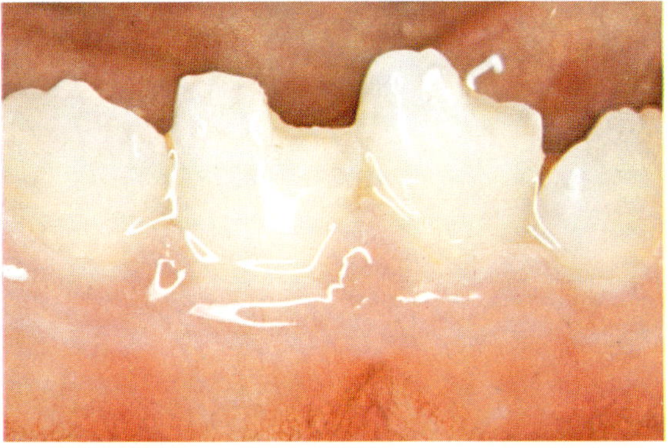

Fig. III-9   Patient S. T. Mandibular anterior fractures can be just as successfully treated as maxillary fractures. The same bevel technique is used in preparing the teeth for acid etching. Mandibular teeth are somewhat more difficult to operate on, because of their smaller size, but the basic technique for restoration is the same as for maxillary teeth.

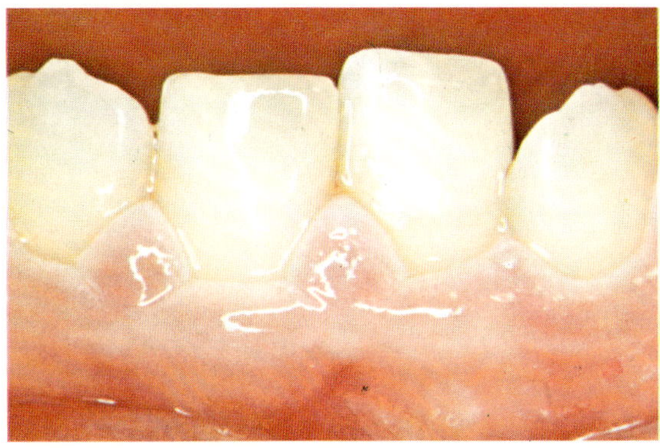

Fig. III-10   Patient S. T. The finished restorations on the mandibular central incisors.

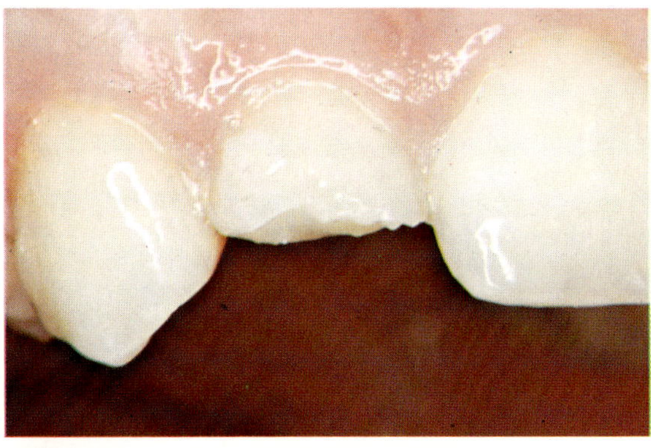

Fig. III-11   Patient C. N. Lateral incisors are not as frequently fractured as central incisors. However a direct blow to a lateral can cause fracture without damage to the adjacent teeth. A fracture of this size will require careful basing with a calcium hydroxide base as in Fig. III-3.

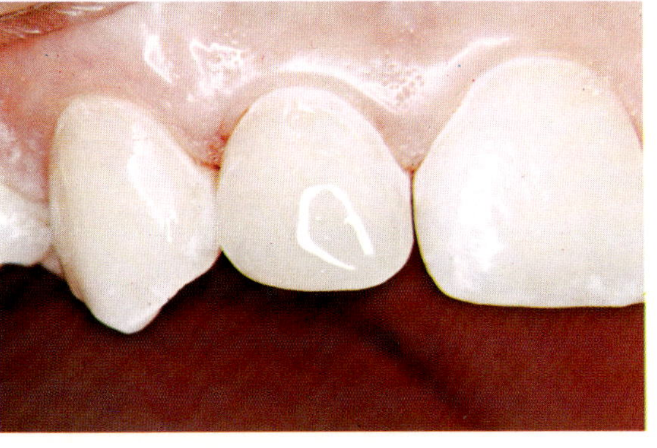

Fig. III-12   Patient C. N. The lateral incisor after restoration and glazing. Care must be taken when glazing to remove excess resin interproximally before polymerization. This is simply accomplished by pulling a Mylar strip through the contact area once or twice.

Fig. III-13   Patient D. S. Teenagers are unfortunately all too frequently seen with stainless steel crowns covering fractured incisors. This is psychologically very traumatic for the child, particularly in adolescence. These crowns are also frequently poorly adapted causing gingivitis and caries. The U-15 scaler could be placed half-way down the labial surface of this crown due to poor adaptation.

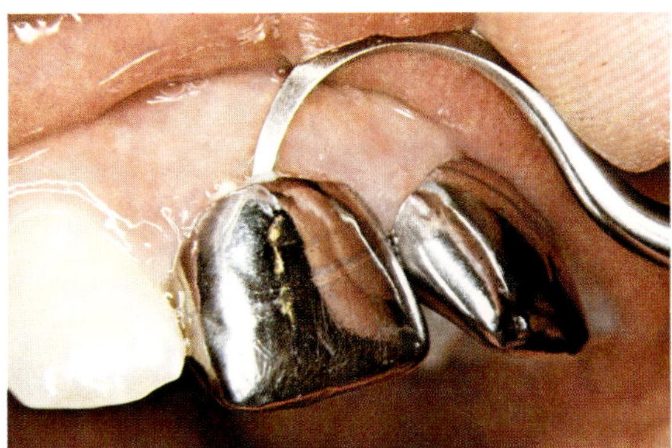

Fig. III-14   Patient D. S. The lingual view of the same teeth disclosed lingual caries at the margin of the stainless steel crown on the left central, (tooth on the left), where the fracture line extended subgingivally and was not covered by the crown. Subgingival fractures are difficult to restore with composite but with careful hemorrhage control and good matrix adaptation it can be satisfactorily accomplished.

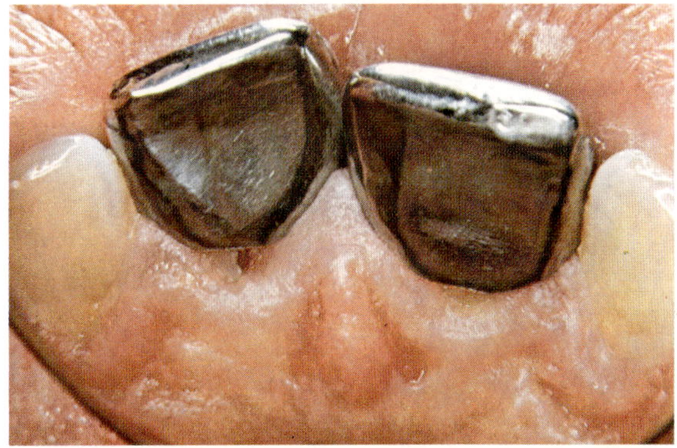

Fig. III-15   Patient D. S. After removal of stainless steel crowns one is sometimes surprised. The upper right central had a very small fracture of the mesio-incisal angle initially. (Part of the original incisal edge is still present). However, in order to fit the crown, the treating dentist had removed a distal slice of the tooth and some labial and lingual enamel which complicated the composite restoration.

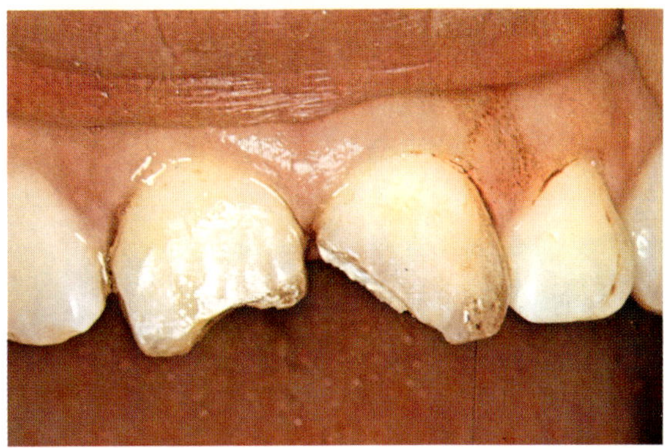

Fig. III-16   Patient D. S. The labial view of the restorations after glazing. The end result is infinitely more esthetically acceptable than the stainless steel crowns. The development of the acid etch technique has eliminated the need for using crowns to protect fractured incisors.

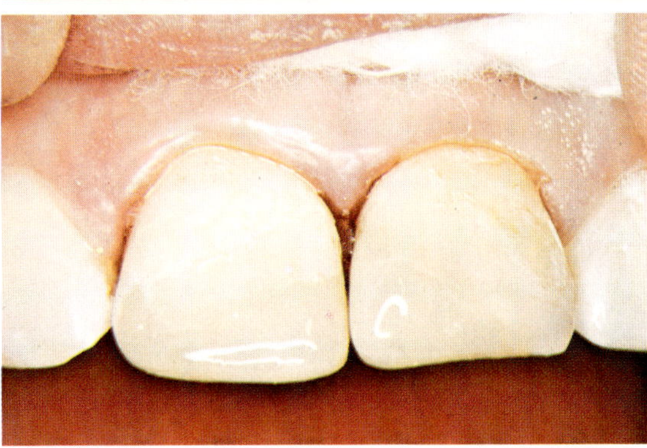

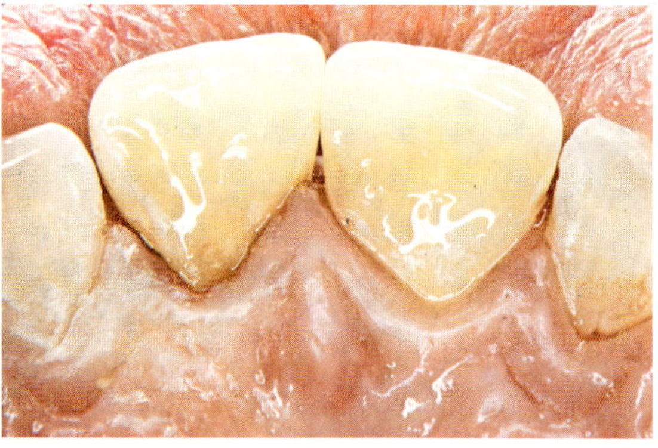

Fig. III-17   Patient D. S. The lingual view of the restorations after glazing. The fracture on the left central (tooth on the left) went subgingivally to the gingival attachment area. After removal of caries, a matrix was formed and composite etched into the lingual (mesial) area first, before the rest of the crown was completed.

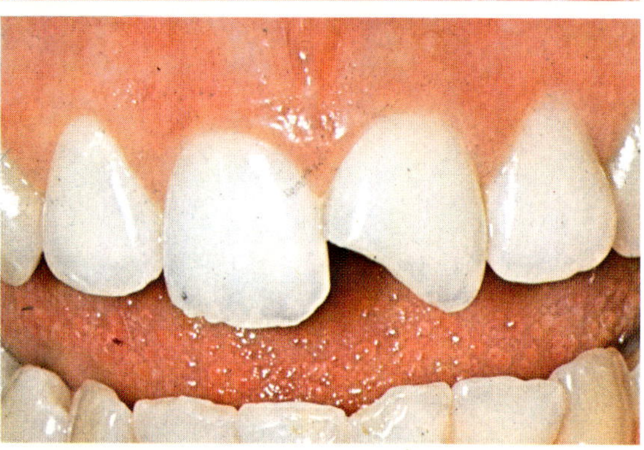

Fig. III-18   Patient B. A. This 16 year old female fractured a central incisor at age 8. She was informed that she would have to wait until her late teenage years for a porcelain jacket crown. Fortunately this was avoided by building up a Nuva-Fil restoration which was glazed with a layer of Nuva-Seal.

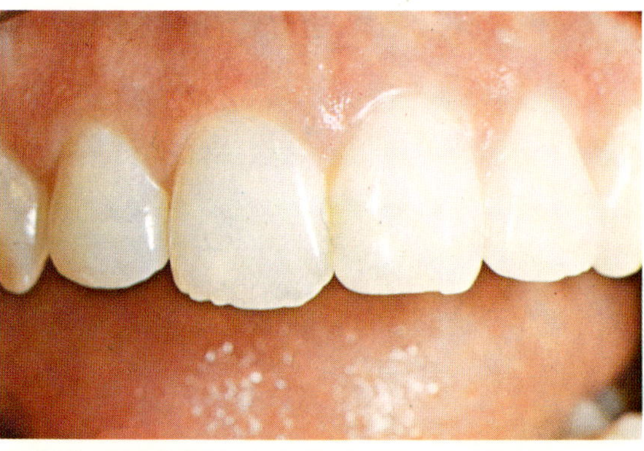

Fig. III-19   Patient B. A. One year after restoration the presence of the glaze layer was clinically detectable. The light reflection on the left central incisor is brightest on the tooth enamel above the fracture line. There is then a wedge-shaped area of no light reflection (no glaze) and an area of dull light reflection where glaze is present.

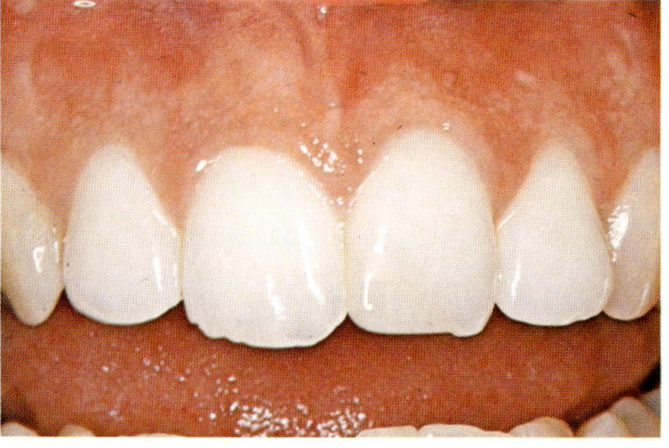

Fig. III-20   Patient B. A. After three years the restoration was clinically acceptable with no deleterious color change or breakdown of the material. The glaze layer was still clinically detectable as a very smooth surface. Tape replicas were taken at each recall for S.E.M. examination of glaze and composite wear on the labial surface.

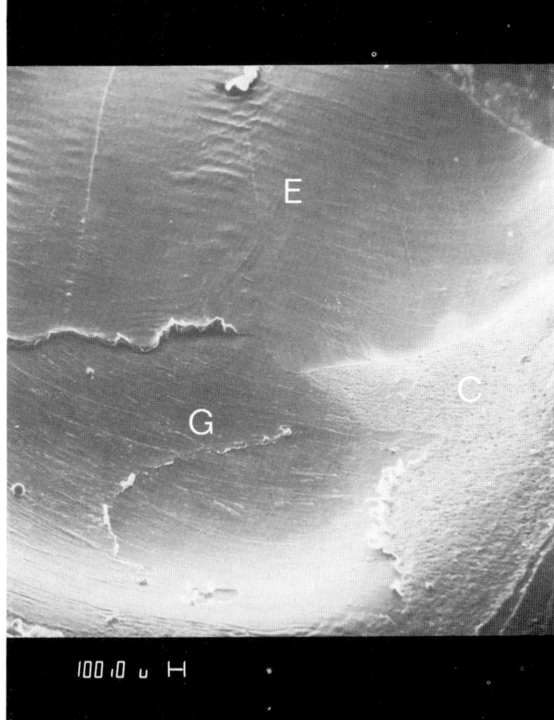

Fig. III-21   Patient B. A. Scanning electron photomicrograph of the negative tape replica of the labial surface of the restored fractured incisor seen in Fig. III-19, one year after restoration. The fracture line extends from approximately two o'clock to the eight o'clock position. E is the enamel surface above the fracture line. C is the exposed composite with no glaze and G is the glaze layer which covers the fracture margin.

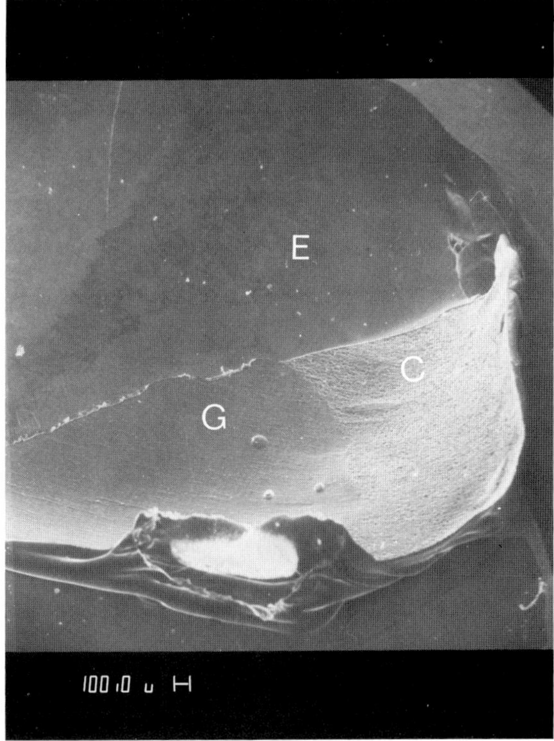

Fig. III-22   Patient B. A. After two years, a new replica was taken. Some wear of the glaze layer can be seen where two small "islands" of glaze are visible. These areas were, at one year, part of the main glaze layer.

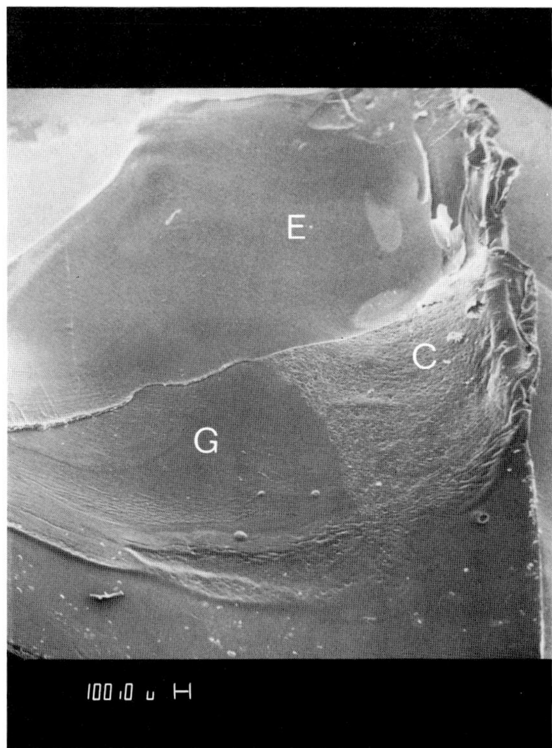

Fig. III-23 Patient B. A. Three years after restoration the "islands" of glaze can be seen to be disappearing as the glaze layer slowly wears down.

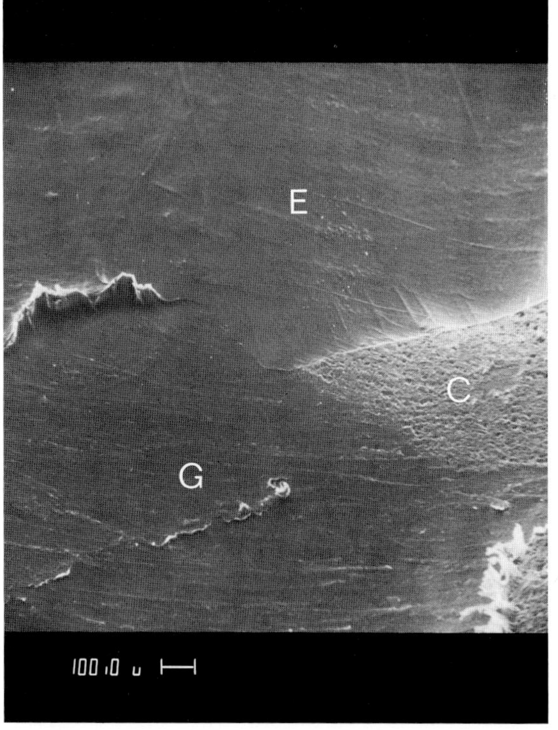

Fig. III-24 Patient B. A. A higher power view of Fig. III-21, the one-year replica. Ignoring the replication artifacts, the area of glaze that comes to a point at four o'clock on the photograph can be compared to the "islands" of glaze formed at two years (Fig. III-25). Note the excellent condition of the enamel/composite margin and the fact that the margin where glaze is present is completely covered, since glaze is bonded to enamel.

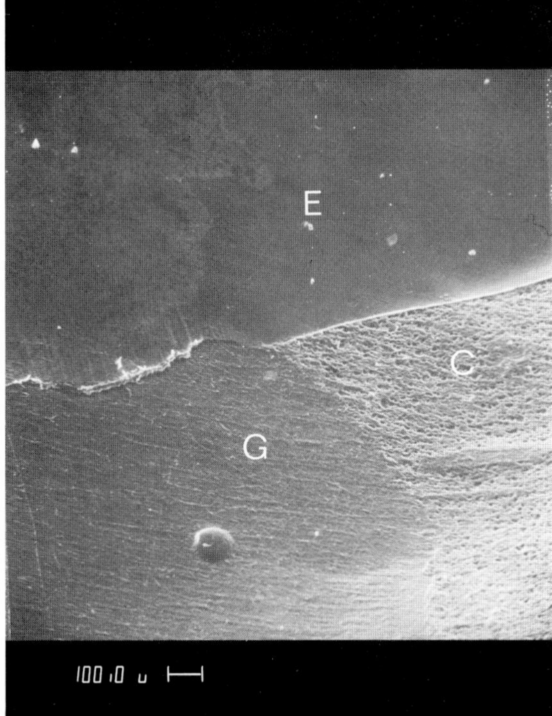

Fig. III-25 Patient B. A. The two-year view at higher power shows the "islands" of glaze that have formed as the original area has worn somewhat. Glaze is still present covering the original fracture margin. The bevel preparation technique leaves a strong margin of composite that is more resistant to breakdown than a feather-edge margin.

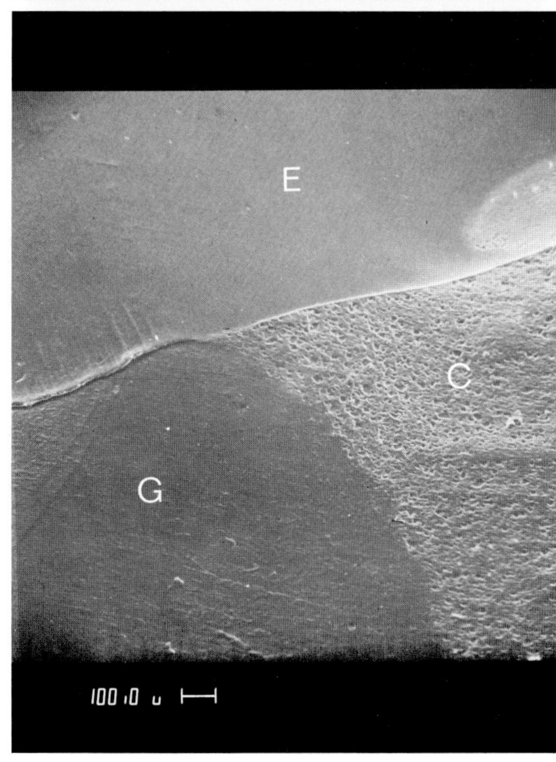

Fig. III-26 Patient B. A. At three years the "islands" are disappearing, although their presence is still detectable. Again note the excellent condition of the enamel/composite margin. No significant breakdown of composite is occurring and glaze is still present over a large area of the restoration.

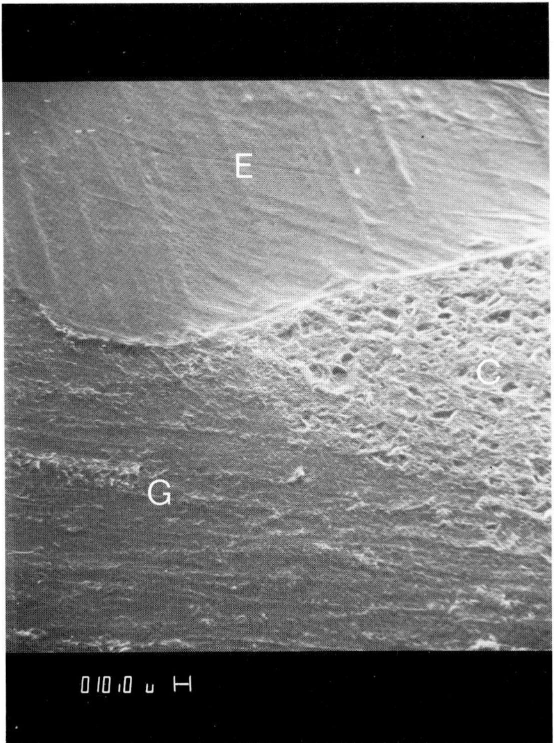

Fig. III-27 Patient B. A. The area where enamel meets composite and glaze is examined under even higher power at one year. The wear of glaze and composite can be compared to the two and three year replicas (Figs. III-28 and 29).

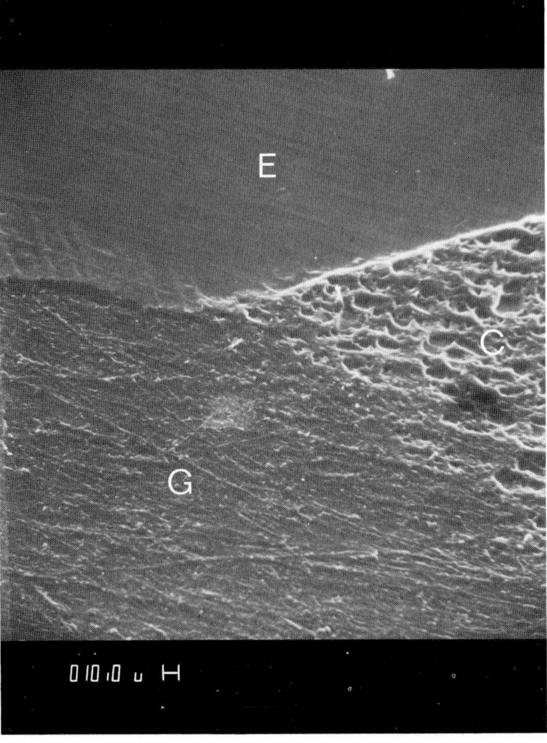

Fig. III-28 Patient B. A. The enamel-composite-glaze interface as photographed on the two-year replica. The composite surface can be seen to be slightly rougher than at one year. The filler particles have become more exposed as the less wear-resistant matrix wears down.

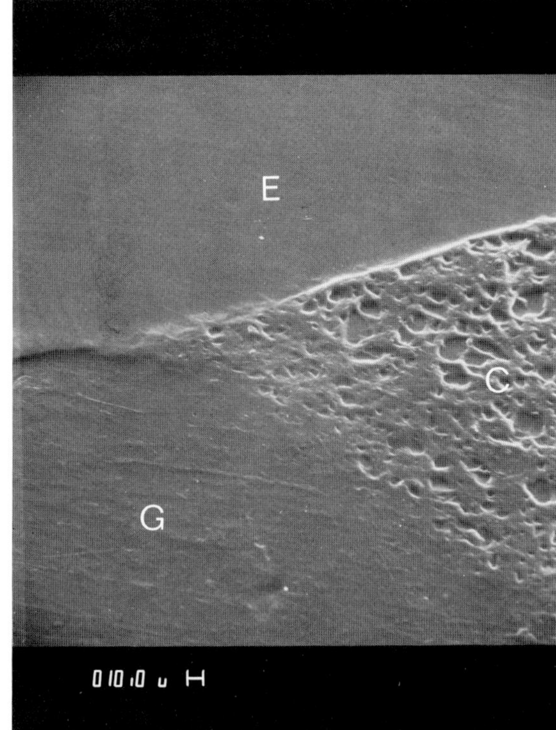

Fig. III-29   Patient B. A. At three years more filler particles are becoming exposed as the glaze wears down at the glaze/composite margin. By picking out filler particle landmarks and comparing with Fig. III-28 the amount of Nuva-Seal wear on the labial surface of a central incisor between two and three years after application can be visualized.

References

1. *Asmussen, E.:*
   Penetration of restorative resins into acid etched enamel. IADR abstract no. 349, February 1977.

2. *Buonocore, M. G.:*
   The Use of Adhesives in Dentistry. Charles C. Thomas, Publisher, Springfield, Illinois, 1975.

3. *Dogon, I. L.:*
   Studies demonstrating the need for an intermediary resin of low viscosity for the acid etch technique. Proceedings of an International Symposium on the Acid Etch Technique, pp. 100–118. North Central Publishing Co., St. Paul, Minnesota, 1975.

4. *Dreyer Jorgensen, K.:*
   The adaptation of composite and non-composite resins to acid etched enamel surfaces. Proceedings of an International Symposium on the Acid Etch Technique, pp. 93–99, North Central Publishing Co., St. Paul, Minnesota, 1975.

5. *Forsten, L.:*
   Effect of different factors on the marginal seal of composites. IADR abstract no. 427, February, 1977.

6. *Jordan, R. E., Suzuki, M., Gwinnett, A. J., and Hunter, J. K.:*
   Restoration of fractured and hypoplastic incisors by the acid etch resin technique: a three-year report. JADA, 95: 795–803, 1977.

7. *Mohammed, H., Schoen, F. J., and Burrell, E. R.:*
   A simple comparative adhesion test method for composite resins. IADR abstract no. 350, February, 1977.

8. *Raadal, M.:*
   Mikroretensjon av plastfyllingsmaterialer paa syreetset emalje. Den Norske Tannlaegeforenings Tidende. 10: 404–413, 1975.

9. *Simonsen, R. J. and Stallard, R. E.:*
   Surface characteristics of composite restorations, IADR abstract no. 314, February, 1976.

10. *Simonsen, R. J.:*
    Acid etch as a preventive technique in dentistry. Chapter 18, in A Textbook of Preventive Dentistry. Caldwell, R. C. and Stallard, R. E. (Eds.). W. B. Saunders Co., Philadelphia, 1977.

11. *Ulvestad, H.:*
    Personal Communication.

Chapter 4

The Acid Etch Technique in Class III and Class V Restorations

It can be stated categorically, that all composite restorations should be placed utilizing the principle of acid etch bonding. The main benefits of etching enamel margins, prior to composite placement, are the maintenance of marginal integrity and the elimination of marginal leakage, in addition to the obviously greatly increased retention.

Preparation

Preparation outline, for acid etched composite restorations, is determined solely by:

1. Extent of caries.
2. Access to caries.

No attention, during preparation, need be paid to the extension for retention. The size and shape of the preparation is basically the end result of caries removal, since prepared, mechanical retention is unneccessary in acid etched composites. The only healthy tooth structure removed is that which has to be removed for access to carious tooth structure. After caries removal, a small bevel is placed all the way around the enamel margin, similar to, and for the same reasons as, the bevel placed on anterior fractures (Chapter 3).
In cases where caries dictates placing a margin on cementum, it may be necessary to cut some small retentive areas on the cementum wall, as etching cementum does not produce the same bonding effect as with enamel. All enamel margins should be etched, even if they comprise only part of the restoration's total marginal length.

Restoration

All exposed dentin should be based with a calcium hydroxide base prior to etching. Etching, and use of the unfilled, followed by the filled, resin follows the identical technique described in Chapter 7, including use of the Centrix C-R syringe for composite placement. The reader can refer to Chapter 3 for comments on the use of the intermediary resin layer, and for the glaze technique.
In, for example, small Class III restorations with tight contact, it may not be possible to re-etch and glaze the restoration. 3M Sof-Lex discs are the polishing technique of choice. The discs are used after contouring the restoration with composite finishing burs, (7901 FG and 7408 FG Midwest American carbide). A Mylar strip matrix provides for a very smooth finish, so use of the composite finishing burs should be restricted to polishing flash from margins. Hopefully, these areas can then be reached with a Sof-Lex disc. The interproximal polishing strips presently available, do not provide as smooth a finish as the Sof-Lex disc. However, improvements in strips, possibly by the Sof-Lex principle, will undoubtedly be available in the future.

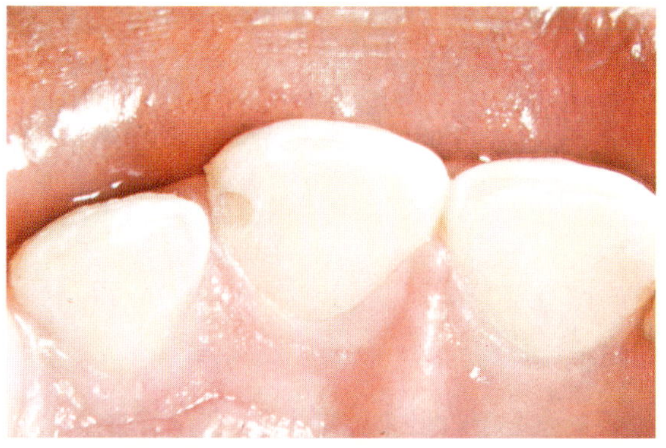

Fig. IV-1 Patient R. S. All Class III composites should be placed utilizing the acid etch technique. Acid etching enables the operator to make minimal preparations, removing only carious tooth structure. No preparation for retention is necessary. All enamel margins should be bevelled. Dentin should be based and the composite placed from a syringe with a Mylar strip matrix.

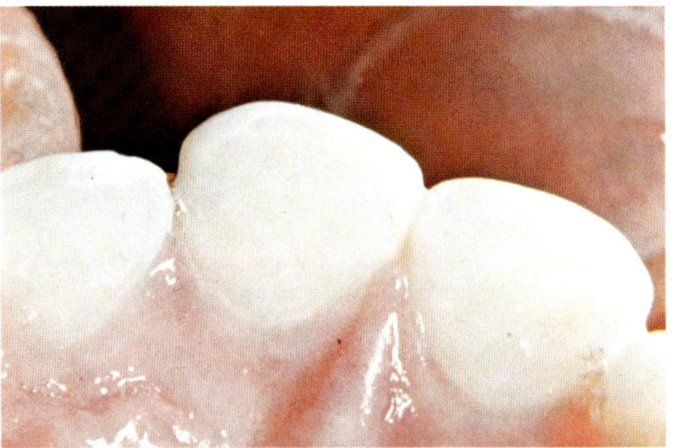

Fig. IV-2 Patient R. S. The finished Class III composite. In the deciduous dentition where diastemas are present it is relatively simple to place a glaze layer on the composite. In the adult dentition it is usually impossible to get a glaze layer interproximally. It is therefore best to rely as much as possible on the Mylar matrix for the finished surface, polishing margins only as necessary for flash removal.

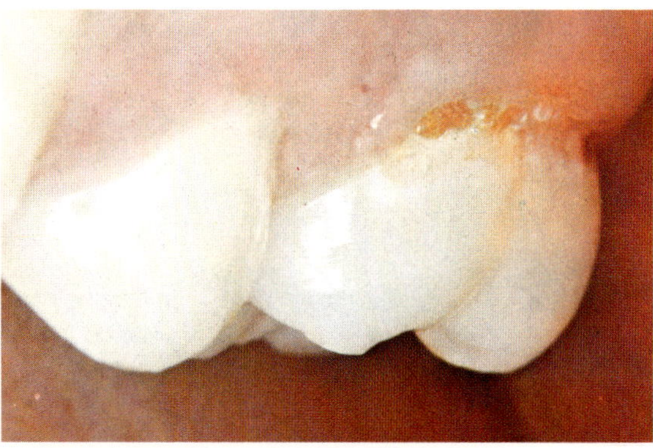

Fig. IV-3 Patient T. J. All Class V restorations with at least one margin in enamel should be acid etched. This will minimize the preparation necessary to removal of carious tooth structure and bevelling of enamel margins. Marginal leakage and secondary caries will be eliminated in acid etched restorations where the correct technique is followed.

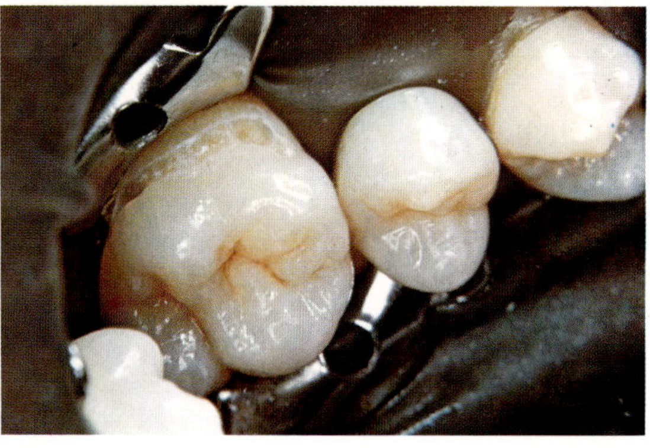

Fig. IV-4 Patient T. J. After placement of the rubber dam the retainer may have to be pushed apically to retract the gingiva from the carious lesion. A medium sized round bur in the slow-speed handpiece is frequently all that is needed for caries removal. The enamel margins are bevelled with a high-speed composite finishing bur or bullet-shaped diamond.

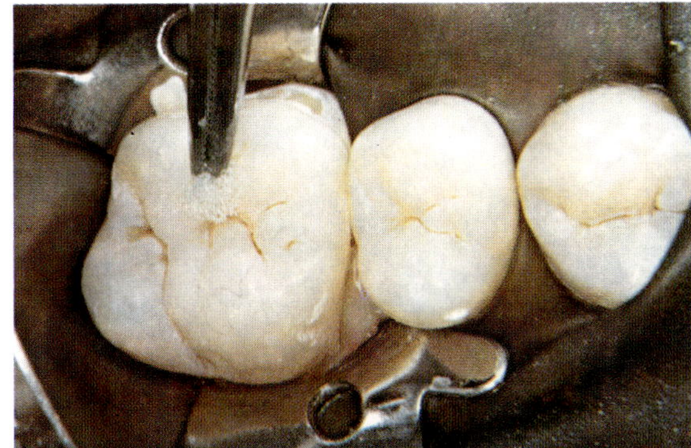

Fig. IV-5   Patient T. J. After basing all dentin with a calcium hydroxide base the enamel margins are etched using the small sponges from the 3M Enamel Bond kits. While the quadrant is isolated under rubber dam, the caries-susceptible occlusal surfaces should be etched for sealant placement.

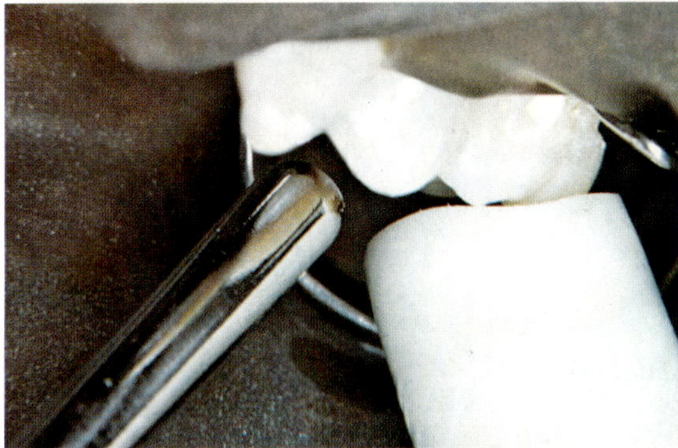

Fig. IV-6   Patient T. J. It is extremely important after etching to thoroughly wash all etched enamel. The excess acid and reaction precipitates must be completely removed. High volume evacuation is essential. The water and/or water spray for washing should be directed at each surface etched for at least 15 seconds before starting to carefully dry the surface.

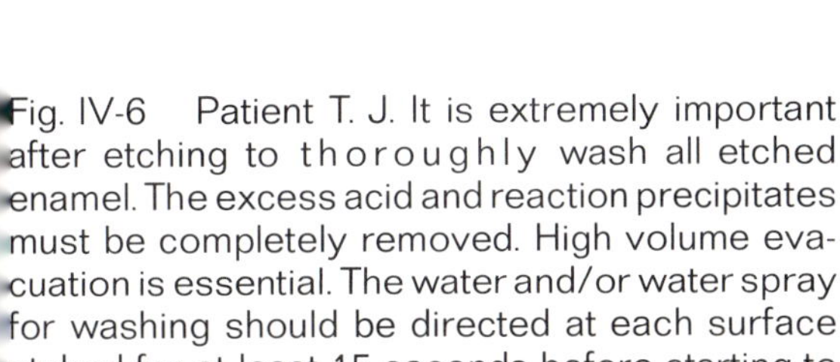

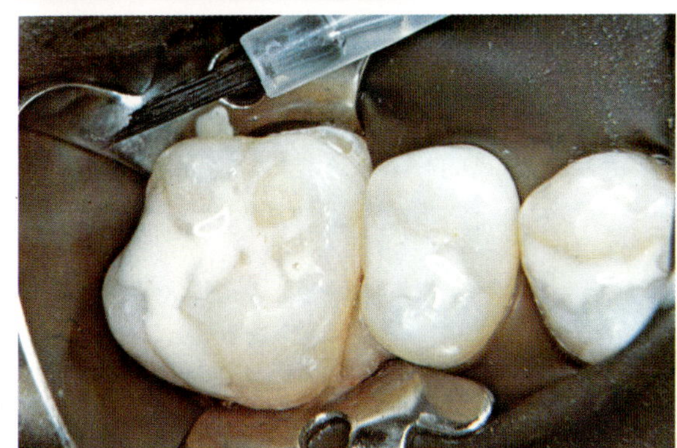

Fig. IV-7   Patient T. J. 3M White Sealant is applied to all the etched occlusal pits and fissures. Enamel Bond (clear unfilled resin) is applied to the cavity preparation and margins immediately before the Concise filled resin is applied with a composite syringe.

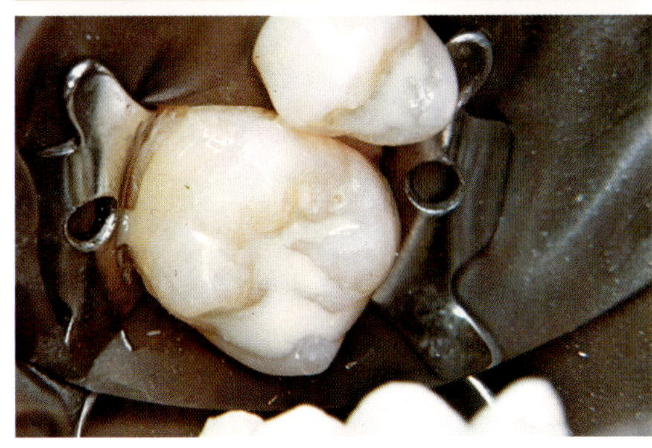

Fig. IV-8   Patient T. J. The filled resin is applied in excess and allowed to polymerize.

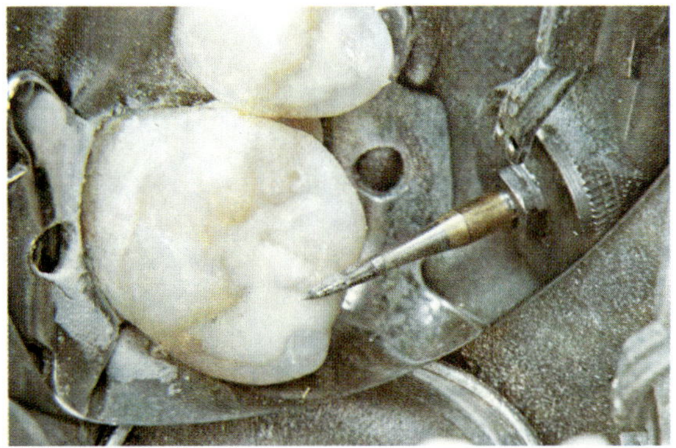

Fig. IV-9   Patient T. J. Approximately four minutes after placement the composite can be trimmed using a high-speed fluted composite finishing bur (7901 FG Midwest American). The high-speed can be used with or without water, although in general when trimming or removing composite it is easier to see the enamel/composite margin if the bur is used dry.

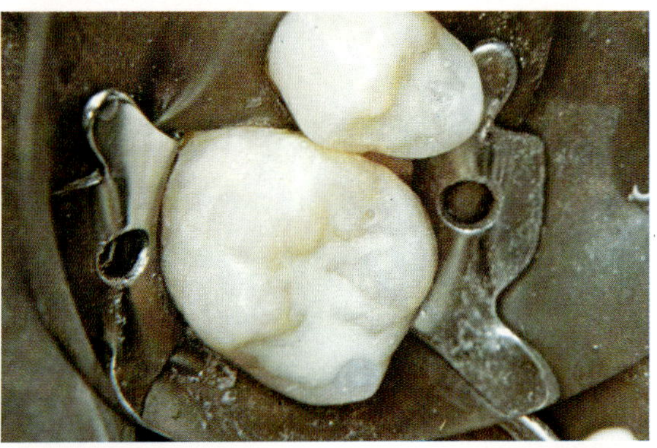

Fig. IV-10   Patient T. J. When the excess has been removed, the restoration can be polished and/or glazed. Before glazing, the margins of the restoration are etched once again and thoroughly washed. The glaze will then bond to enamel and the composite, sealing off all the margins of the restoration.

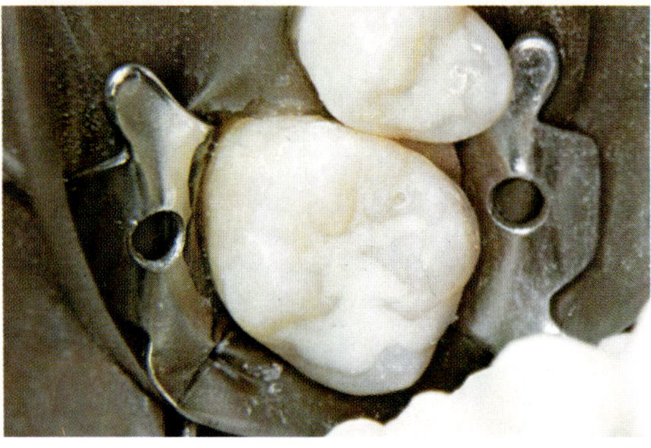

Fig. IV-11   Patient T. J. The glaze layer is allowed to polymerize for two minutes and then the excess unpolymerized surface layer of unfilled resin is wiped off.

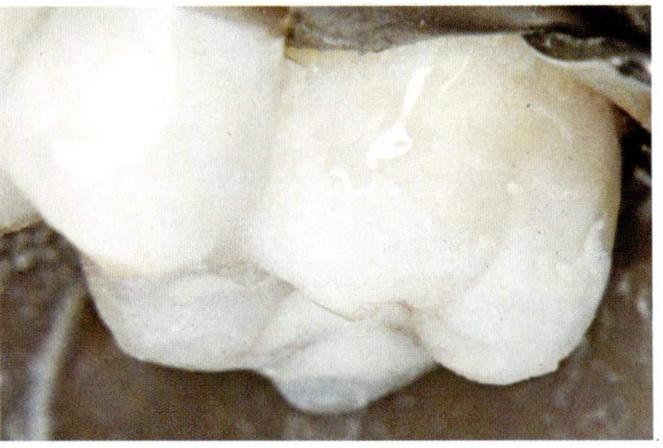

Fig. IV-12   Patient T. J. The finished restoration viewed from the buccal.

Chapter 5

Developmental Defect Restoration

The restoration of developmental defects, along with the restoration of fractured incisors, is a most rewarding aspect of the acid etch technique. Many people have deep complexes about their physical appearance. Teeth, particularly upper anterior teeth, play a large part in the overall impression other people get of one's appearance.

It is gratifying, indeed, to have at our finger tips a technique, so simple to master and execute, that can give such joy to people previously burdened by unsightly defects of their teeth.

The technique steps are basically the same as already described in Chapters 2 and 3.

1. Wash
2. Prepare (if necessary)
3. Etch for 60 seconds
4. Wash and dry thoroughly
5. Apply intermediate unfilled resin layer
6. Apply filled composite resin
7. Trim and polish
8. Re-etch
9. Glaze

For details of the technique, refer to Chapters 2 and 3. To avoid repetition, only those factors unique to each particular type of restoration, will be discussed.

Restoration of peg laterals

Peg laterals are ideal for acid etch restoration, providing a large area of enamel for bonding. The step-by-step procedure is detailed in the legends to Figures V-1 to 7.

For applying the composite (Fig. V-4), there are basically two choices of matrix. The first is a plastic crown form, selected for size and trimmed to fit the peg stub. The disadvantage of using a crown form matrix for composite addition, is that peg laterals tend to have a rather small cervical circumference. This makes adaptation of the crown form in this area very difficult.

The alternative matrix is the Mylar strip seen in Figure V-4. It may appear to be a somewhat "untidy" composite restoration at this stage, but the important cervical area of composite, is flush with the tooth on the mesial, lingual and distal surfaces. This leaves excess only on the easily accessible labial surface.

The 7901 FG Midwest American carbide finishing bur is excellent for trimming down excess composite. The 7901 is also thin enough so that it can be introduced into the gingival sulcus if subgingival flash has to be removed (Fig. V-5).

If subgingival trimming has irritated the tissue enough to cause hemorrhage, a piece of gingival retraction cord can be placed in the sulcus (Fig. V-6), to obtain hemostasis prior to glazing.

Restoration of hypocalcification defects

Unsightly defects in the enamel can be rapidly masked with composite resins. Some operators prefer to veneer over the defects. This, however, leaves an unnatural contour to the labial surface, and it should be avoided, if possible.

White hypocalcification defects are frequently very shallow and can be simply removed by discing the surface layer of the enamel away. If this fails, a "scoop" of enamel is removed, with a tear-drop shaped high-speed diamond, to allow for space for the composite. The darker (and more difficult to mask) the defect, the deeper the scoop, taking care to always stay within the enamel layer if possible (Fig. V-10).

The scooped-out enamel area is etched and then unfilled, followed by filled resin, of the desired color shade, is added. If the defect is a great contrast to natural tooth color, it may show through the composite. When this can be anticipated beforehand, a layer of special opaque composite is placed in the deepest portion of the "scoop" preparation. Composite of the desired exterior shade is then simply added to the opaque layer after polymerization.

Re-etching and glazing is desirable for most hypocalcification restorations. Figure V-11 shows a case with the labial restoration half glazed. The other half is polished with 3M Sof-Lex discs to study the wear characteristics of disc polish versus glaze layer over time (Figs. V-21 and 22).

Restoration of anterior diastema (shape alteration)

Two cases of anterior addition for closure of a diastema are seen in Figures V-15 to 20.

The mesial portion of each central incisor is, in turn, etched and composite added using a Mylar strip matrix (Fig. V-19).

In a matter of a few minutes, a problem that may have bothered someone for years, can be solved. The basic shape of teeth can be similarly altered.

Other defects, such as tetracycline stain, fluorosis stain and areas of decalcification as a result of orthodontic banding, can be treated similarly. The masking of tetracycline stains is probably the most difficult and challenging defect to hide. Usually, in these cases, the complete labial surface is covered with composite after removal of a surface layer of enamel.

Glaze finish as opposed to disc finish

Figure V-21 is a scanning electron photomicrograph of a replica taken of the labial surface of Figure V-11. The replica was taken at the 6-month recall and shows the margin between the enamel surface (E), the Sof-Lex polished composite (C) and the glaze (G). It should be remembered that both Figures V-21 and 22 are negative replicas, thus the glaze appears on the left of the photograph, whereas Figure V-11 shows the glaze to be on the right half of the restoration.

The large areas of roughness seen in the glaze are from bubbles within the glaze that burst after polymerization, exposing areas of the polished composite underneath. The original experimental glaze, (3M Co.), was full of bubbles, and this caused some problems. Later experimental glazes, however, have been de-gassed, eliminating the problem.

Figure V-21 shows clearly the effect of re-etching and glazing over the margin. Where glaze covers the margin, the margin is completely protected against breakdown and marginal leakage (see also Figs. III-21 to 29).

Figure V-22 shows a higher power view of the glaze/composite interface. The glaze can be seen to be very smooth. While the Sof-Lex disc polished composite is also very smooth compared to other polishing techniques, it is not as smooth six months after application, as the glaze finish. These scanning electron photomicrographs are part of a continuing study into the comparative smoothness and wear of a glaze layer, compared to a disc polished layer. Tentative 6 and 12-month results indicate that a bubble-free glaze is smoother at application, 6 and 12 months than the best presently available polishing disc, the 3M Sof-Lex disc.

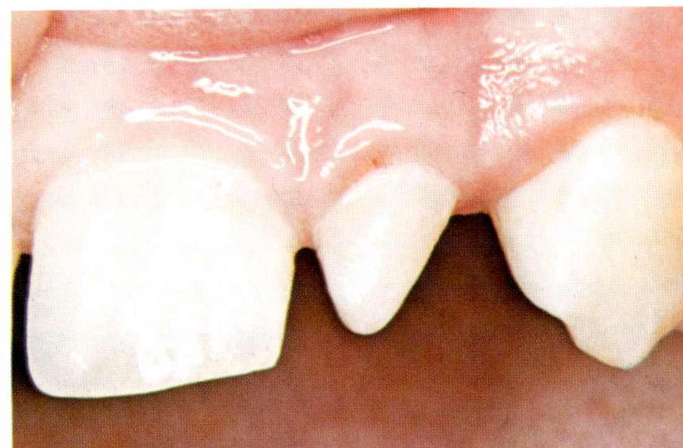

Fig. V-1　Patient K. B. Developmental defects, such as peg laterals, can be simply corrected with composite resins and the acid etch technique. A peg lateral such as this can make a child extremely self-conscious.

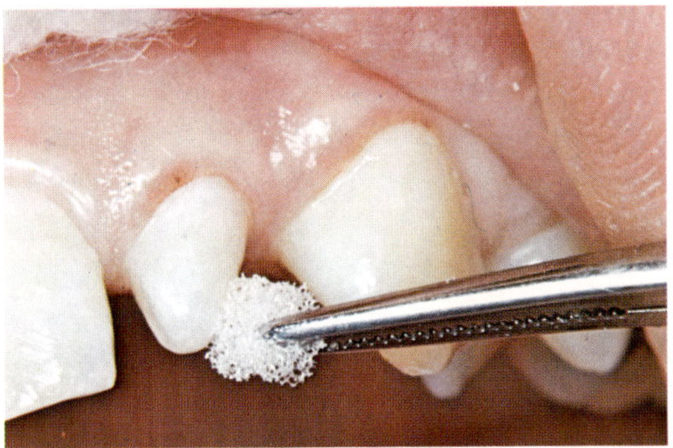

Fig. V-2　Patient K. B. The complete stub can be etched after cleaning the enamel surface. The 3M Concise Enamel Bond kits contain small sponges suitable for applying the 37% orthophosphoric acid. The acid should be applied to all the enamel surfaces needed for bonding. Fresh acid should be continually re-applied for one minute.

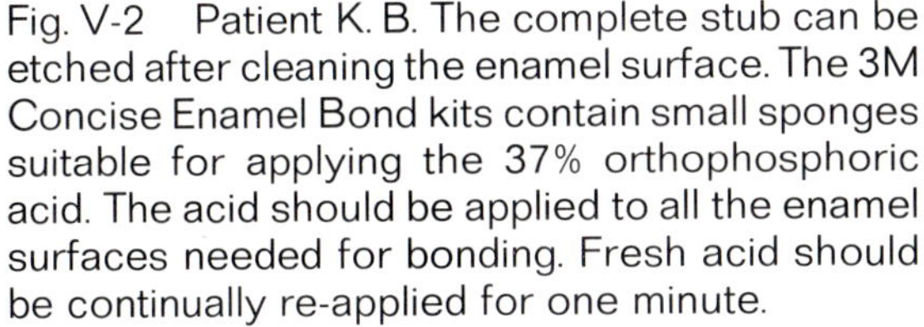

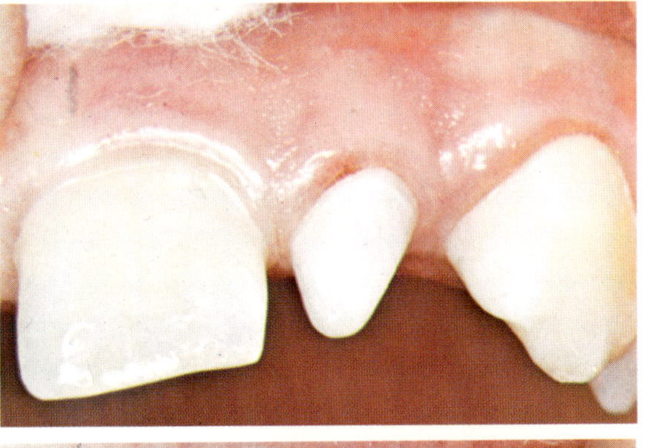

Fig. V-3　Patient K. B. After thorough washing and drying the enamel takes on the characteristic frosty white appearance of etched enamel. Washing away the acid must be done very thoroughly to ensure removal of all excess acid and reaction precipitates. Immediately prior to Mylar strip matrix placement, a layer of unfilled resin (3M Enamel Bond) is placed over the complete area of etched enamel.

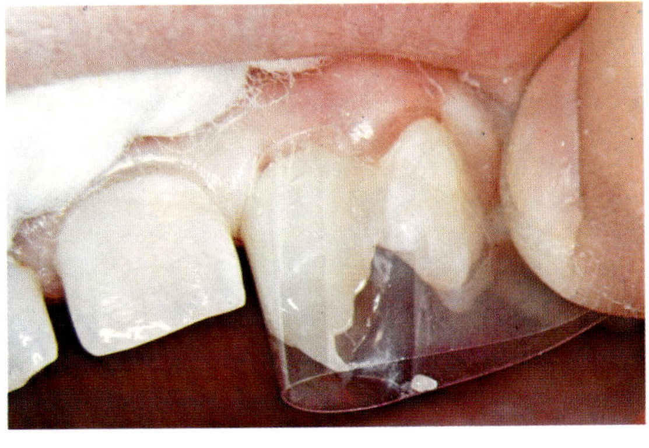

Fig. V-4　Patient K. B. Most peg laterals have a very constricted cervical circumference making cervical adaptation of plastic crown forms rather difficult. An alternative method is to use a Mylar strip as a matrix and let the composite polymerize in excess. The excess material can be trimmed down using a composite finishing bur in the high-speed handpiece.

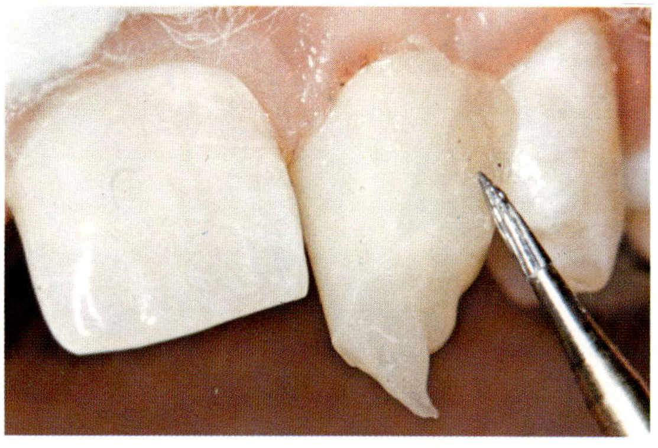

Fig. V-5   Patient K. B. The fluted composite finishing bur is excellent for trimming down the excess composite. Diamonds can be used for gross removal and discs for the final polish prior to glazing.

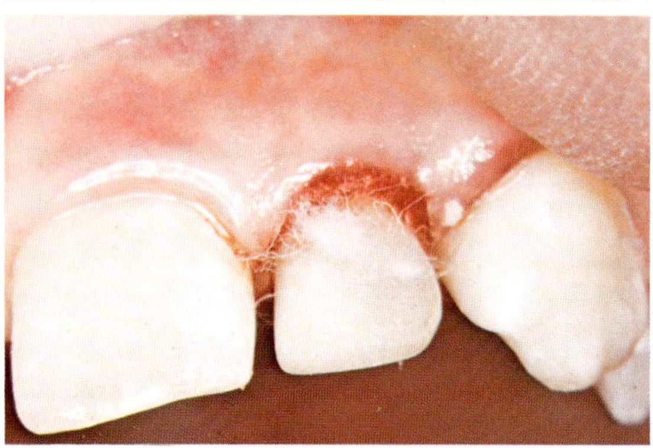

Fig. V-6   Patient K. B. After subgingival trimming of excess composite (the composite is feather-edged preferably away from the gingival crest), it may be necessary to place some gingival retraction cord into the sulcus to initiate hemostasis prior to glazing.

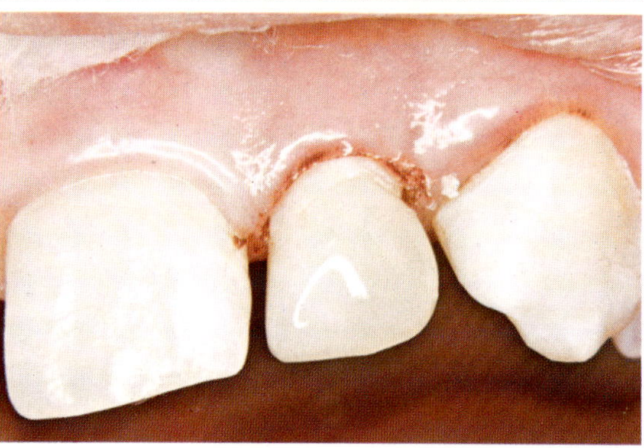

Fig. V-7   Patient K. B. The cord is removed and the restoration glazed. The beauty of the acid etch system is its reversability. If, after completion, the patient is not satisfied with the appearance of her new tooth, the composite can be removed leaving the peg lateral as it was previously.

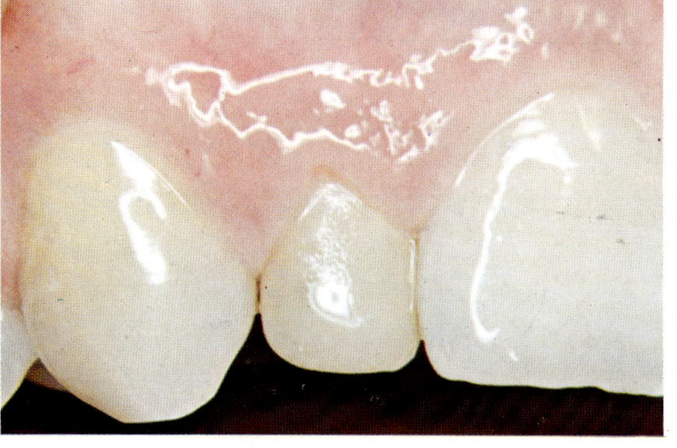

Fig. V-8   Patient S. M. This composite-restored peg lateral is 32 months old. The material seems to have yellowed somewhat, its color approaching that of the cuspid rather than staying the same as the central incisor as it was originally. This is, however, of minor significance when one considers the dramatic improvement in appearance that was gained.

Fig. V-9   Patient M. D. Hypoplastic defects are common and sometimes are so unsightly that patients are willing to have the teeth crowned to hide the defect. Using composite resins and the acid etch technique these defects can now be quickly masked. Some operators prefer to veneer over such defects, but the change in the contour of the labial surface that results is undesirable.

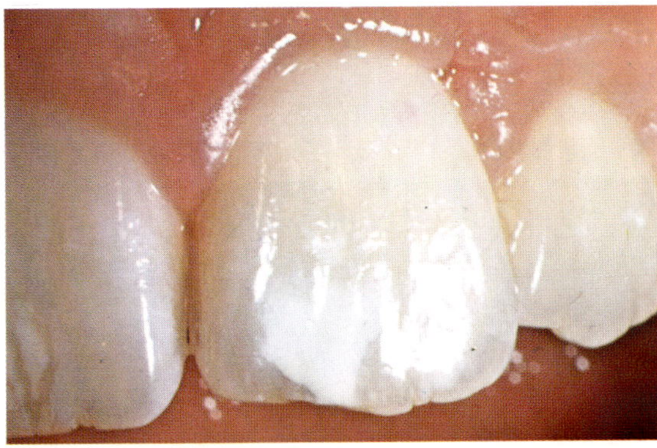

Fig. V-10   Patient M. D. Some white hypoplastic defects are so shallow that simply discing them will remove the discolored area. In this case, however, the defect was through the complete depth of enamel. Thus an area of enamel about 0.5 mm deep at the center was scooped out using a diamond. The area was etched about 2 mm beyond the edge of the preparation.

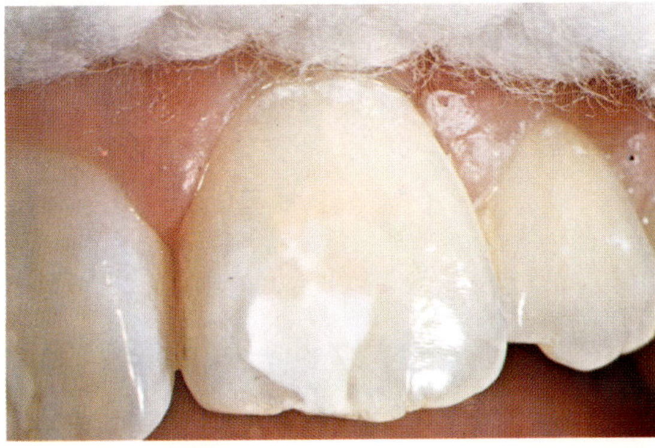

Fig. V-11   Patient M. D. After addition of the correct shade of composite this particular restoration was finished in two different ways to be able to study the surface wear over time. (Figs. V-21 and 22). One half of the composite was polished with 3M Sof-Lex discs, the other half was glazed. If the defect shows through the composite as some dark stains may, a layer of opaque Concise can be placed under the final color.

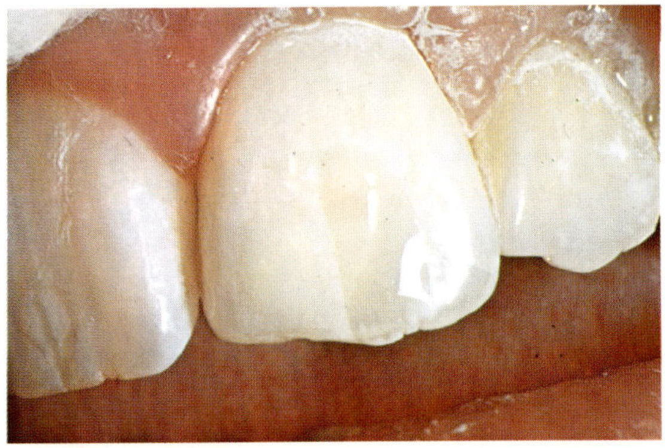

Fig. V-12   Patient M. D. The 6 month recall photograph of Fig. V-11. It is not possible on this photograph to tell the difference between the two differently polished halves. However, after a replica is taken, a difference can be clearly seen under S.E.M. (Figs. V-21 and 22).

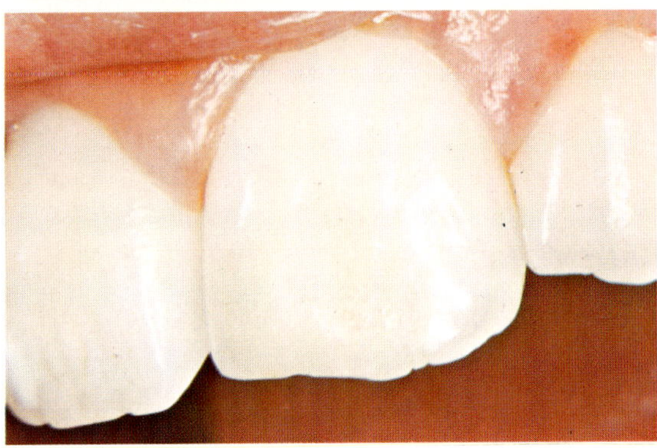

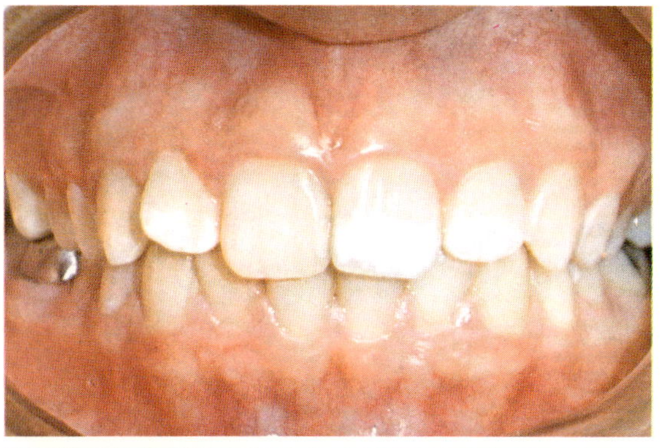

Fig. V-13   Patient D. M. This teenage girl was anxious to have her left central incisor crowned. However she was persuaded to accept an attempt at correcting the problem utilizing acid etched composites. The same technique as used in the previous case was followed.

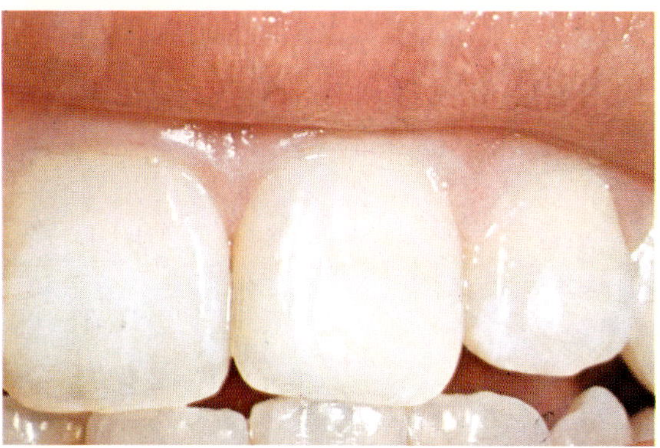

Fig. V-14   Patient D. M. The restoration was completed in 15 minutes with an excellent result.

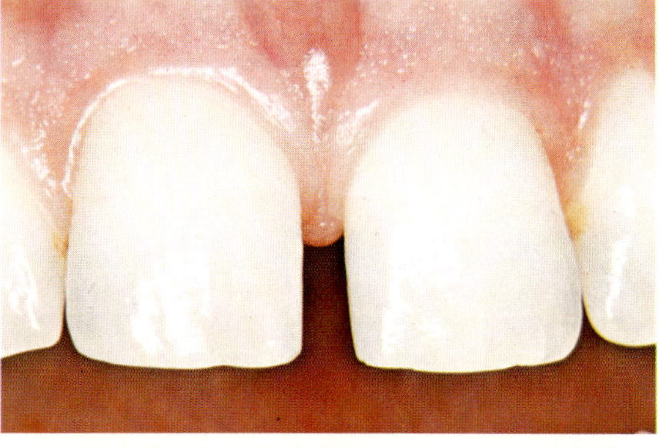

Fig. V-15   Patient B. S. Diastemas of this kind are seldom successfully treated orthodontically without permanently anchoring the centrals together to prevent relapse. It is very simple to etch the mesial enamel and add some composite using a Mylar strip matrix.

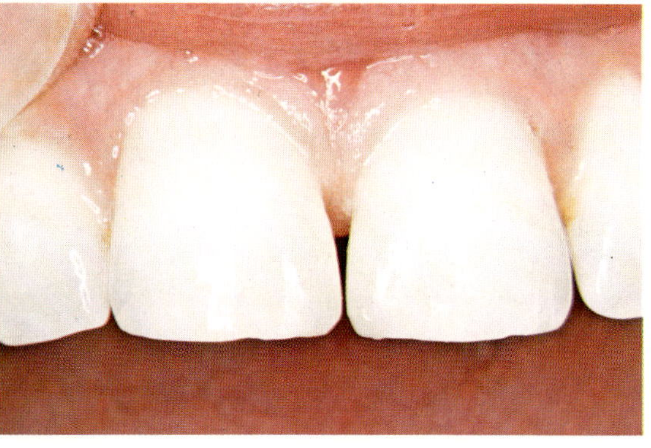

Fig. V-16   Patient B. S. The finished double mesial addition. Nothing irreversible has been done to the teeth and patients are invariably extremely happy with the result.

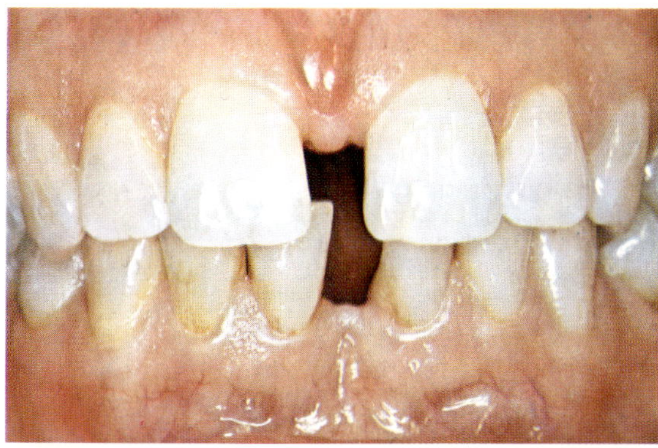

Fig. V-17   Patient B. F. In this extremely severe diastema one cannot hope for a perfect correction. Closing the diastema completely with composite would result in some very oddly shaped centrals. A compromise must be aimed for to achieve an improvement in the situation.

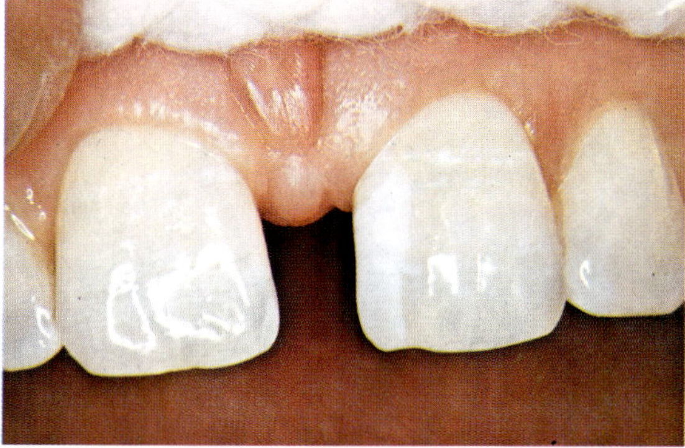

Fig. V-18   Patient B. F. The mesial portion of the tooth requiring composite addition is etched. About ¼ to ⅓ of the labial and lingual surfaces are etched.

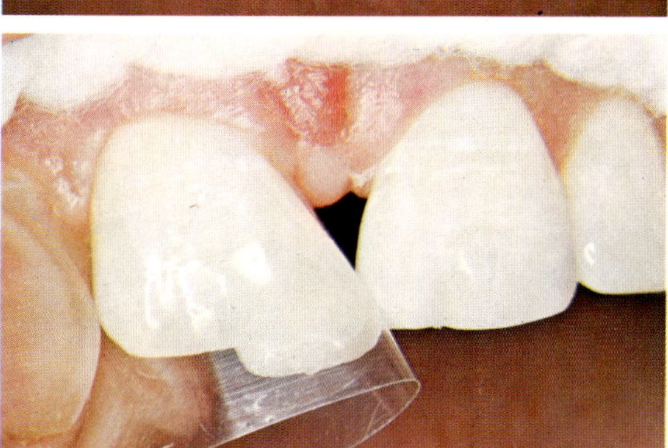

Fig. V-19   Patient B. F. The Mylar strip is angled away from the tooth as it rests on enamel at the gingival crest mesially. Composite is added on top of an unfilled resin layer. In this case the left central has been completed and the right central is having composite added.

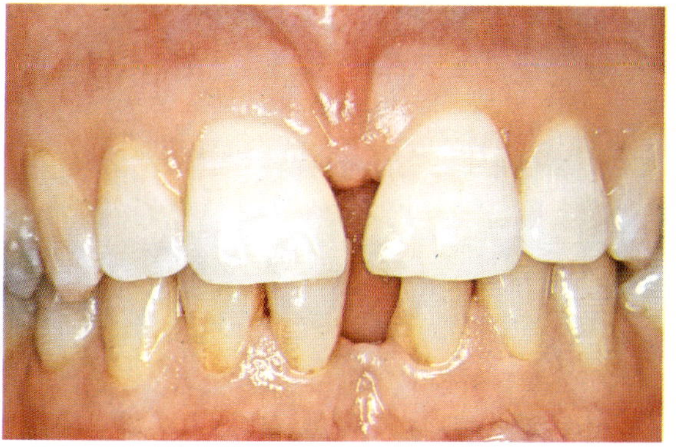

Fig. V-20   Patient B. F. The end result left a small diastema to avoid over-contouring the centrals.

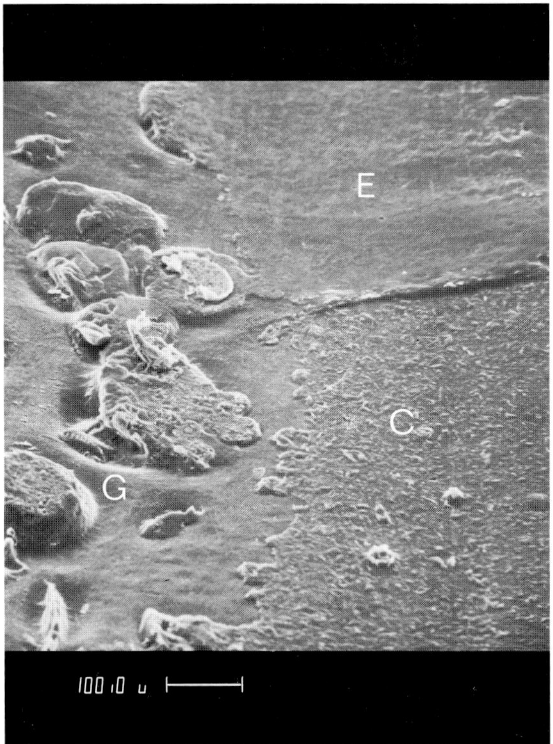

Fig. V-21   Patient M. D. This replica of the surface of Fig. V-12 is shown under S.E.M. six months after finishing the restoration. The glaze layer (G) on the left can be seen to be pitted with bubbles which extend to the surface of the filled resin underneath. The glaze can be seen to cover the margin between composite (C) and enamel (E).

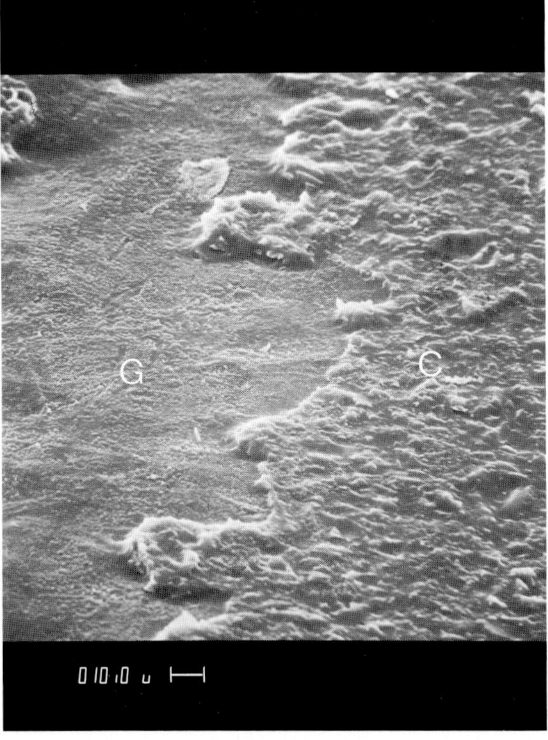

Fig. V-22   Patient M. D. This higher power view shows the glazed surface on the left (G) and the filled resin surface on the right (C). After six months the glaze layer is smoother than the filled resin which was polished with the best discs presently available, (3M Sof-Lex). The bubble problem in the glaze was solved in a later experimental glaze.

Chapter 6

The Acid Etched Bridge

Soon after it became clear that the acid etch bond, when properly applied, was an extremely strong bond, investigators started utilizing denture teeth, bonded in place of missing teeth, for temporary bridges.

Several ways of improving the technique have been applied over the years the technique has been in use. As different investigators use the technique and develop their own improvements, it is certain that a very satisfactory method of quickly providing an inexpensive and esthetic bridge, with almost no abutment teeth preparation, will be adopted by the dental profession.

The minimal expense in manufacture means that this kind of bridge can be readily employed in cases where doubtful prognosis of abutment teeth, (whether from periodontitis, caries or trauma), would have contraindicated the placement of a conventional bridge. Little or no tooth preparation of abutment teeth means that, should the bridge fail, one can always progress to a more radical (based on amount of tooth preparation necessary) gold bridge. As in other uses of the acid etch technique, in cases of failure, one is only back where one started. Properly completed, however, the procedure to be described results in very few failures.

It was not known during initial attempts with acid etch bridges, how long they would last. Just as with a conventional bridge, it still cannot be forecast how many years of service one can expect. The improvements in the technique to be described here, lead to the belief that one can, on the average, expect several years of service from such bridges.

Initial attempts using denture teeth resulted in anterior bridges lasting approximately two years, (Figs. VI-1, 11 and 16). *Ibsen* and *Neville*, in an excellent chapter entitled, "Adhesively Bonded, Fixed-Bridge Prostheses", quote a life expectancy of 6–18 months for bridges utilizing resin denture teeth pontics.[2] Using the technique described here, life-expectancy can be estimated to be at least two years, and probably much longer. With further advances in composite resin materials and technique, the life-expectancy of these bridges can only improve.

Techniques for Anterior Bridges

Acrylic denture teeth, with mechanical retention cut into the lingual surface for composite resin material, were successfully used in initial attempts at acid etch bridges.[1,2,4] *Buonocore*[1] describes cutting a mesiodistal retentive groove on the lingual surface and then roughening all surfaces of the pontic to be utilized in bonding prior to applying a drop of methyl methacrylate to these surfaces. The conventional technique of applying unfilled, and then filled, resin is followed.

Buonocore also describes a method which this author prefers at the present time, namely of using the filled composite resin for the pontic. Initial attempts at anterior bridges had one weak point—namely the "bond" between the composite resin and the acrylic resin denture tooth. Almost to the month, two years after application, many of these bonds were fracturing (Fig. VI-1, 11, 17). No fracture in bonds between resin and enamel have ever been seen, but the mechanical (lingual) "bond", (and whatever could be obtained chemically with the use of methyl methacrylate), was apparently the weakest link in the restoration. Thus, it was decided to make the pontic out of composite resin and obtain a chemically united uniform material. This has been successfully achieved and, although it is more difficult to obtain an esthetically pleasing labial surface with composite, it is felt that the increased life span expectancy justifies the slight esthetic disadvantage.

In certain cases of multiple root fractures, evulsions or periodontal extractions, the tooth itself, after root removal, pulp tissue removal and canal sealing, can be utilized as the pontic. This provides for an excellent esthetic result (Fig. VI-23).

Since all three techniques, (use of denture tooth, composite or natural tooth pontic), are basically the same, a detailed description of the method utilizing a composite resin pontic, which is the best presently available technique, will be given. A good description of acid etch bridges using acrylic denture teeth can be found in *Buonocore's* book[1].

Technique for composite resin pontic bridge

Very little preparation of abutment teeth is necessary. The surface adjacent to the missing tooth must be clean. Should there be an old Class III or larger restoration present, it should be removed, so that clean, fresh enamel margins are present. Enamel margins should be bevelled to remove any loose enamel rods and to give enamel prisms their correct orientation for ideal etching.

The first step in making any bridge is the taking of impressions for study models. This model is used in the adaptation of the pontic to the ridge, prior to the patient's appointment time.

A clear plastic crown form of the correct size is filled with a mix of the desired color shade composite resin (Fig. VI-3). The crown form is removed after polymerization, and the pontic is adapted to the model. A glaze layer is then applied to all of the pontic area that will be in slight contact with the gingiva, providing a perfectly smooth surface to minimize plaque accumulation (Fig. VI-4).

Rubber dam isolation is usually contraindicated in the placement of these bridges. In cases where rubber dam was used, it was frequent that the pontic was not accurately placed on the ridge. If a gap is left between pontic and ridge, it will become an area of food collection and irritation for the patient.

After cleaning and drying the surfaces to be etched, 37% phosphoric acid is applied to one of the abutment teeth (Fig. VI-5). The etch is carried onto about ⅓ of the labial surface and ½ of the lingual surface. This gives ample retentive area. The amount of retentive area used will depend on the amount of stress the pontic tooth is expected to bear. In general the principle is followed of using as little labial retention as possible and as much lingual retention as necessary.

A small amount of unfilled resin is then applied to one corner of the pontic and polymerized to hold the pontic in place for a check of positioning prior to final bonding (Fig. VI-6). If the pontic is not in the desired position adjacent to the abutment tooth, the bond is simply broken and the procedure repeated. If an autopolymerizing system, such as the 3M Concise System is used, (as it is here) a small amount of Universal Paste can be mixed with half a drop of Catalyst Resin. This will give a very fast setting mix which is desirable for a temporary placement set, while holding the pontic between thumb and forefinger, being careful not to touch and contaminate the adjacent etched enamel surfaces.

If the temporary placement is satisfactory, the pontic can then be finally bonded in place using a layer of unfilled, and then filled, resin, feather-edged onto the labial and lingual surfaces of the abutment teeth (Fig. VI-7). The material will form a mechanical bond to the abutment teeth and a chemical bond to the composite pontic. According to *Joos*,[3] the chemical bond between fresh resin polymerized on top of previously set resin, provided the surface of the previously polymerized composite is freshly cleaned, will be between 50%–100% as strong as had the material been polymerized all at one time.

After polymerization, the composite is trimmed down to give as esthetic embrasures as possible without compromising the strength of the bond more than necessary. The lingual surface, since it is not of esthetic importance, can be left smooth with as much composite as is necessary, providing occlusion is not compromised (Fig. VI-8). The final strength of this bridge will depend on the inherent strength of the composite resin used. After polishing down and forming the desired anatomy, a re-etch of marginal enamel and glaze is utilized as previously described (Figs. VI-8 and 9). Figure VI-10 shows the completed all-composite pontic bridge that was made to replace the 2 year-old acrylic denture pontic bridge.

Wire support

In many cases, particularly where more than one pontic unit is necessary, or where previous restorations consume large areas of the adjacent abutment tooth, it will be of benefit to place a wire running through the bridge for added strength.

It is a simple procedure to incorporate a wire within the composite pontic and leave the ends embedded into the mesial or distal preparations of the abutment teeth. If no old preparations exist for the wire in abutment teeth, a small ledge can be cut in the outer enamel layer, or the wire can simply be contoured to blend into the tooth anatomy and bonded to the enamel.

A two year old case of an anterior bridge, with pontics replacing two missing central incisors, is seen in Figure VI-11. Cracks appeared between the composite resin and the acrylic denture teeth pontics after 26 months. The patient had been taking no special precautions to protect the bridge during this time. The pontics were removed (Fig. VI-12), and some all-composite pontics were made, utilizing two clear plastic crown forms, with mesio-incisal corners cut out to provide a continuous band of composite. In addition, a .032" wire was placed through the crown forms, and thus within the composite (Fig. VI-13). After glazing the gingival areas (Fig. VI-14), the pontics were bonded into place (Fig. VI-15).

Although many of the bridges made with acrylic denture teeth broke down after two years, the case seen in Fig. VI-16, where an upper right lateral has been replaced with an acrylic denture tooth, has been in function for 30 months.

In the case of posterior bridges, where occlusal forces are far more severe, a wire is almost obligatory to help withstand stress. Old MO or DO restorations can be removed and the wire so formed to lie within the abutment teeth, which are then restored with composite resin, acid etching all margins. In the case of virgin abutment teeth, a quick check of the occlusion will tell if any tooth preparation is necessary. If abutment teeth marginal ridges are in occlusal contact, a round diamond bur can be used to remove just as much enamel as will allow a wire (usually .032" wire is used) to cross the ridge and lie in the central groove.

Initial attempts at posterior bridges were also

made utilizing denture teeth with no wire support (Fig. VI-17). Surprisingly, perhaps, the replacement of single bicuspid teeth was just as successful as with incisor teeth. The weak link again, was between composite resin and denture tooth. Without wire support, this "bond" seemed to start breaking down at about two years of use in most cases. With the use of a wire support and composite resin pontics, it is felt these bridges can remain functional for many years (Figs. VI-19 to 22).

Wear on the resin occlusal surfaces is the main problem with these bridges. Until resins are developed with greater wear resistance, it will be necessary to add resin to occlusal surfaces every two years or so. This is simply accomplished by removing the surface resin layer and adding fresh resin to the clean surface of the old resin. In most cases, it will also be desirable to freshen up, and re-etch, enamel margins prior to the addition of resin.

Figure VI-22 shows a posterior composite and denture tooth bridge 28 months after placement. A wire support and an old MO amalgam, (removed and replaced with composite), were utilized for greater strength. Part of the wire support is seen on the surface of the first molar, where occlusal grinding at placement removed the covering composite.

As mentioned earlier, the natural tooth is frequently an excellent pontic. In this case (Fig. VI-23) of periodontal loss of a lower anterior tooth, the tooth was stored in a humid environment during healing of the extraction site. After root removal and grinding-in to adapt to the new gingival contours, the crown apex is sealed using composite (which should then be glazed). The original tooth is splinted into place, utilizing the 3M Concise Enamel Bond System. The case in Figure VI-23 has been in function 24 months. The mandibular right lateral incisor had to be extracted for periodontal reasons. The resulting splinted bridge leaves the patient looking exactly the same as before. An additional benefit is the added support given to the periodontally weakened central incisor.

It is impossible for many dentists to justify the preparation of virgin abutment teeth to replace a missing tooth. The acid etch technique provides a means by which satisfactory replacement bridges can be made with minimal or no preparation of adjacent abutment teeth. The advantages of the service rendered to the patient, in replacing a tooth with minimal preparation of adjacent teeth, outweigh the possible longer-term benefits of the conventional, but more radical, fixed gold/porcelain bridge.

The acid etch technique for bridges is still in its infancy. Improvement in materials and techniques will undoubtedly lead to a greater share of the fixed prosthodontic market for this technique. Until that time, it is felt justifiable to carry patients through, with little expense and minimal destruction of healthy tooth structure, with the technique here described. Each time such a bridge needs to be replaced, the new results will be better than the previous ones as improvements in technique and materials are incorporated. Even if the acid etch bridge has to be replaced every two years, (which is unlikely with the improvements already made in the technique), it is certainly justifiable to offer the patient this option. Preservation of tooth structure, thus leaving all options for future treatment open, must remain the highest priority.

The number of ways the acid etch technique can be utilized for fixed bridges, is limited only by the ingenuity and willingness to experiment of the practitioner. Certainly, many patients who would not otherwise be treated can have inexpensive and functional bridges placed. Long-term clinical investigative results will be necessary before it will be known if the procedure is cost-effective. There is no doubt now, however, that a realistic alternative technique to conventional fixed prosthodontics is available.

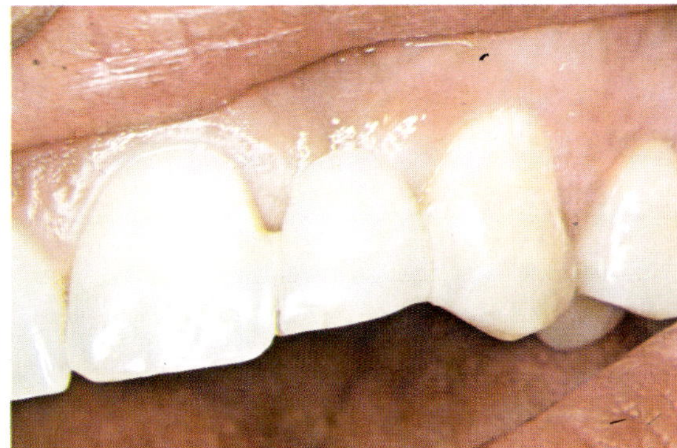

Fig. VI-1   Patient P. K. This acrylic resin denture tooth was bonded to the central incisor and cuspid for 24 months before failure. The patient had previously been wearing a "flipper" partial to replace the missing lateral. Failure of the bridge came as a result of breakdown at the composite/pontic tooth interface. This area is the weak link in all such bridges utilizing acrylic denture teeth as pontics.

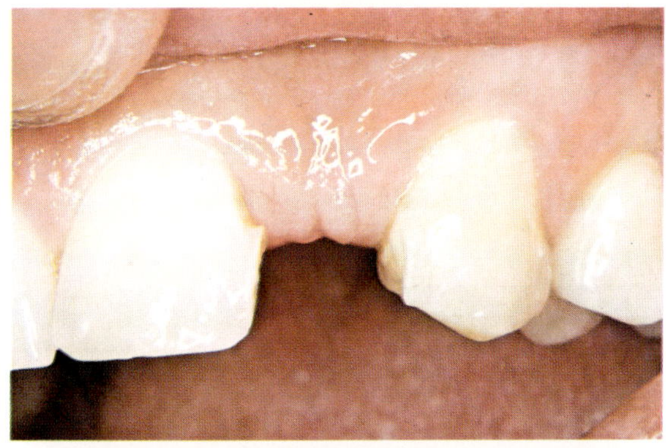

Fig. VI-2   Patient P. K. After removal of the pontic the composite bonded to tooth enamel was still present, confirming the strength of the acid etched bond. However, as in all techniques, the end result is only as strong as the weakest link, and the inherent strength of the materials will determine the strength of the bridge.

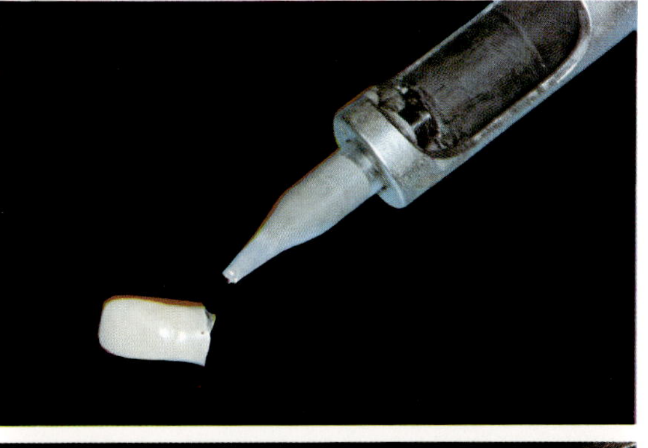

Fig. VI-3   Patient P. K. Since many bridges made with acrylic denture teeth were breaking down at about two years, it was decided to eliminate the weak link by excluding the denture pontic. Instead pontics were made of pure composite resin. The composite pontic would then chemically bond to the composite resin used to bond the pontic to the adjacent teeth. A clear plastic crown form is filled with composite.

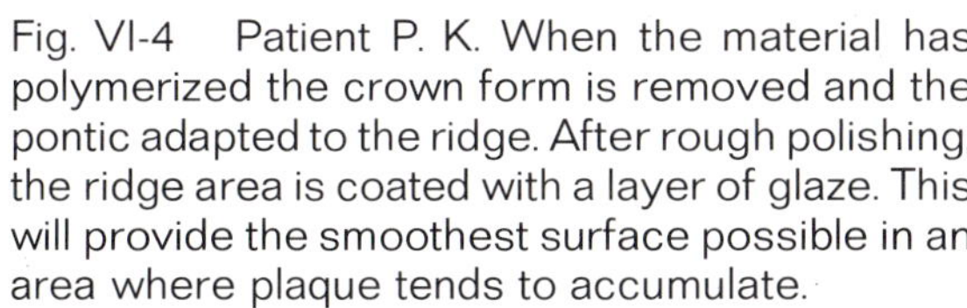

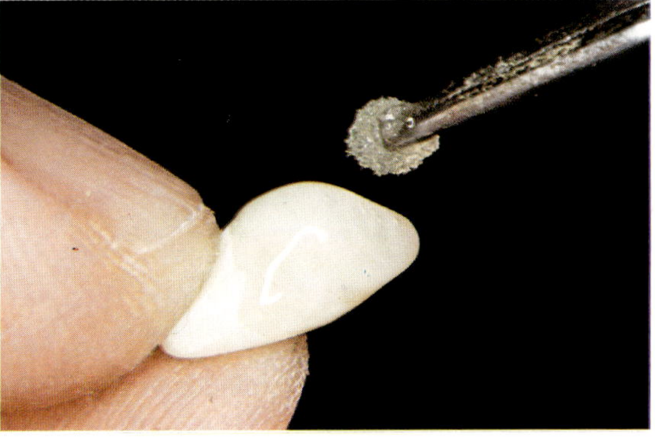

Fig. VI-4   Patient P. K. When the material has polymerized the crown form is removed and the pontic adapted to the ridge. After rough polishing, the ridge area is coated with a layer of glaze. This will provide the smoothest surface possible in an area where plaque tends to accumulate.

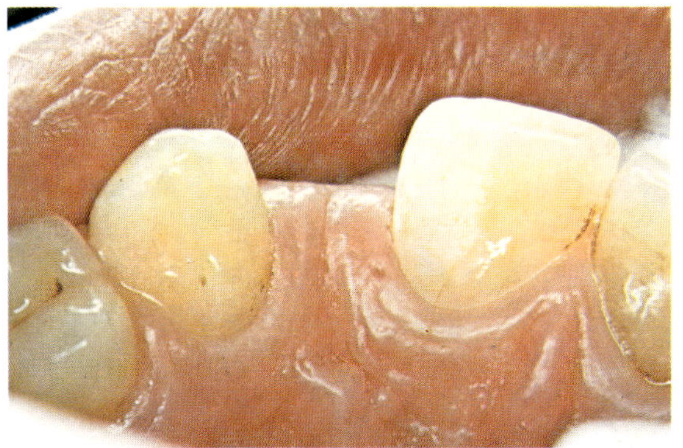

Fig. VI-5   Patient P. K. The old composite bonded to tooth enamel was removed and the teeth cleaned. It is easier to make one bond at a time. In that way it is possible to concentrate on following the technique accurately without being rushed into doing two bonds at once. About one-half of the adjacent tooth can be etched, thoroughly washed and dried. The enamel will have a frosty-white appearance after etching.

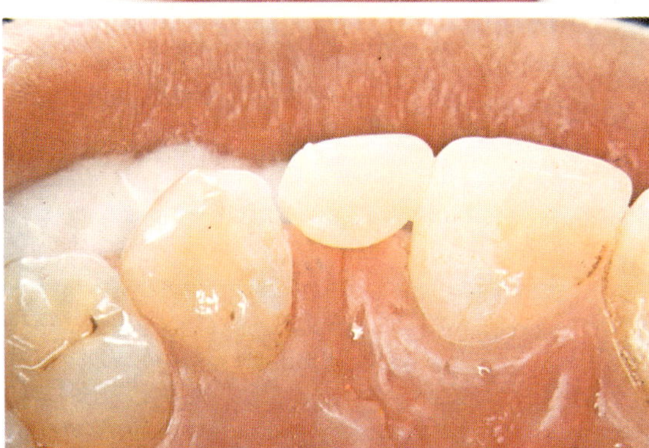

Fig. VI-6   Patient P. K. The pontic tooth is placed into position and held while one drop of unfilled resin is applied interproximally. After polymerization the position of the pontic is checked. If an adjustment is desirable the bond can be easily broken at this stage and the procedure repeated. When the pontic is perfectly aligned, the other abutment tooth can be etched and prepared for resin bonding.

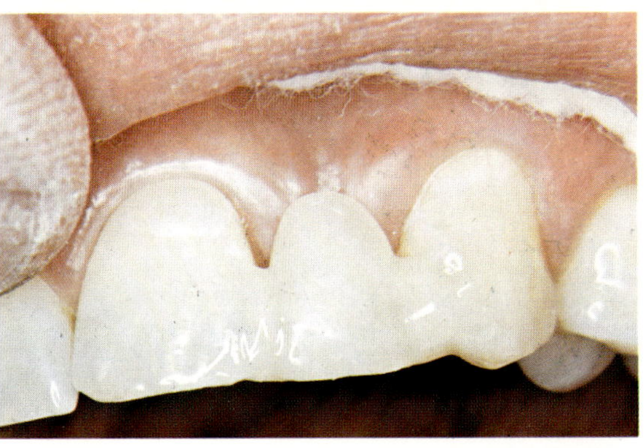

Fig. VI-7   Patient P. K. A thin layer of unfilled resin (3M Enamel Bond) is applied over all etched enamel and pontic bonding areas. This will assure optimal "tag" formation for retention. The filled resin (3M Concise) is then applied, using a composite syringe (Fig. VI-3), to all the interproximal areas labially and lingually.

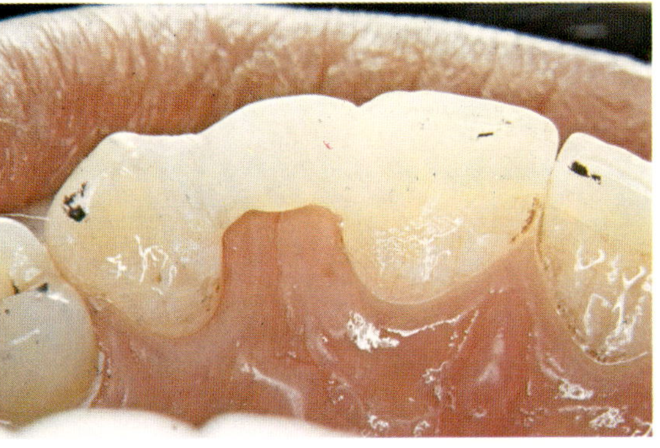

Fig. VI-8   Patient P. K. Using the composite finishing burs all excess composite is removed. The occlusion is checked with articulating paper to be sure the pontic is just slightly out of occlusion. The adjacent enamel is then re-etched about 2 mm beyond the composite margins in preparation for glazing.

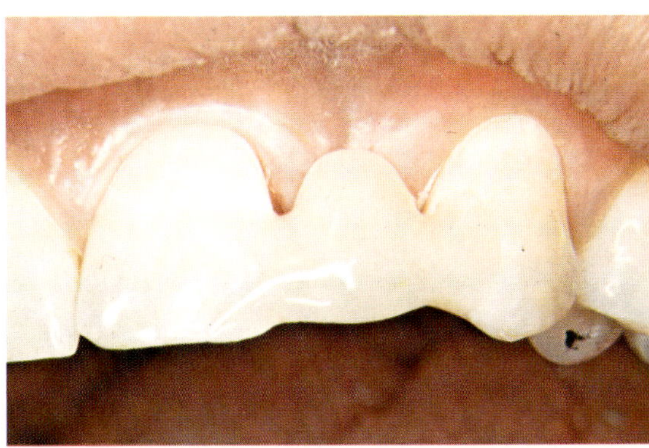

Fig. VI-9   Patient P. K. The glaze layer is applied liberally and flowed beyond the composite margins to seal all margins by bonding into adjacent etched enamel. More contour could be given to interproximal embrasure areas than was done in this case, but each time composite is removed the overall strength of the total unit is reduced. For insurance, as much resin as possible should be left in place.

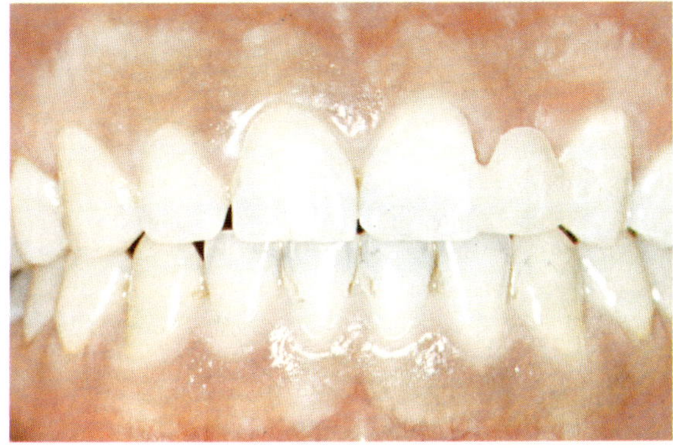

Fig. VI-10   Patient P. K. Full mouth view of the case (Figs. VI-1 to 9). The patient has excellent dental health and both teeth adjacent to the missing maxillary left lateral are caries and restoration free. It is very hard to justify removal of tooth structure from such healthy teeth to replace a missing tooth. The acid etch technique gives us a means of replacing missing teeth with no removal of tooth substance.

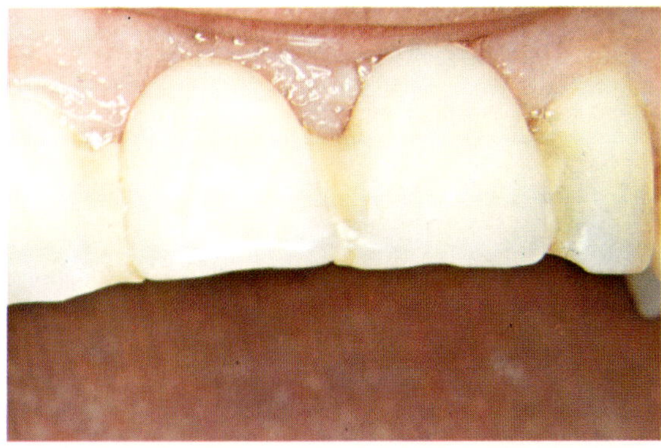

Fig. VI-11   Patient J. F. This acid etched bridge was also functional for a full two years before breakdown was observed at the composite/pontic interface. This bridge replaced both central incisors and had a wire lingually to strengthen the two pontics. The patient stressed at two year recall that he was very happy with the bridge and did not "baby" the teeth at all. Discoloration of the composite can also be seen.

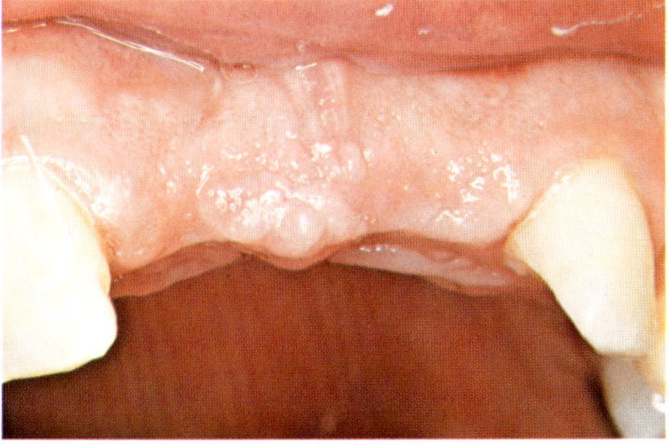

Fig. VI-12   Patient J.F. After removal of the bridge the composite was removed from the adjacent teeth, one of which had an old Class III restoration that was also removed. The gingival tissues appear to tolerate well the placement of such bridges as there is here no sign of inflammation or hyperplasia after two years.

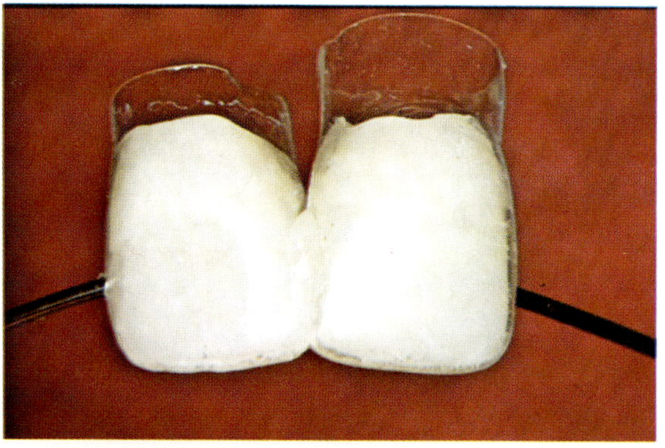

Fig. VI-13 Patient J. F. New pontics were made by bending an arch wire to the curvature of the anterior maxilla. The wire was placed through two clear plastic crown forms and they were both filled with Concise. The mesial contact area of both crown forms had been removed to allow composite from each crown to join.

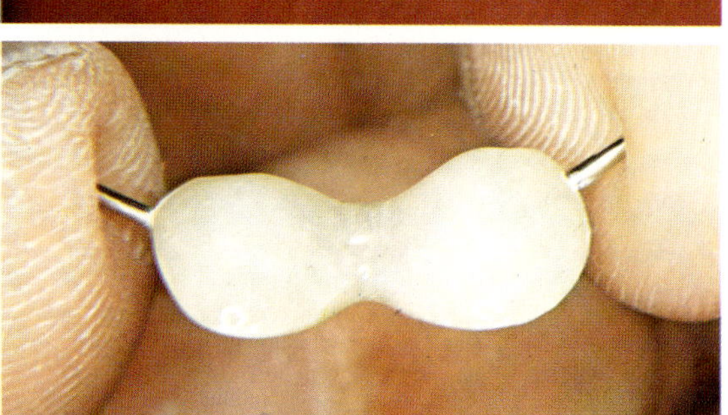

Fig. VI-14 Patient J.F. The pontics were trimmed, polished and the gingival contact area glazed. The wire is cut off so that the end can either rest within the Class III preparation, or just be bonded to the lingual enamel. Sometimes a small ledge can be cut in the lingual enamel where the wire can rest thus strengthening the bridge against occlusal forces.

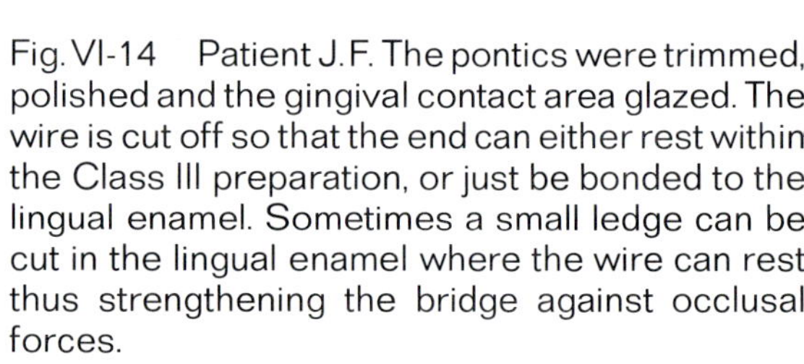

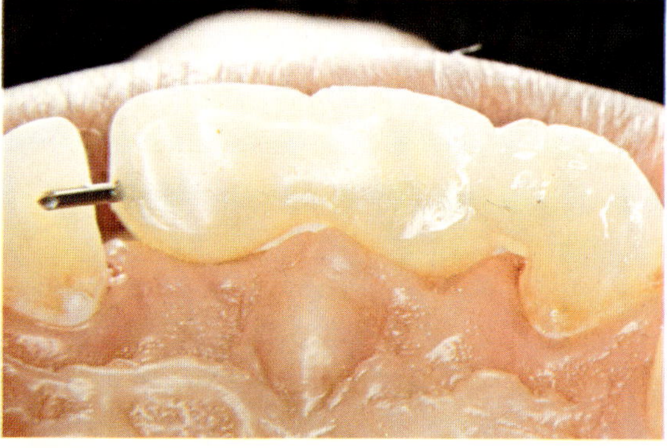

Fig. VI-15 Patient J. F. A lingual view after bonding of one side. The smooth glazed surface on the pontics is apparent. To minimize the chances of contamination of etched enamel, etching of the second abutment tooth is not carried out until the first bond has polymerized.

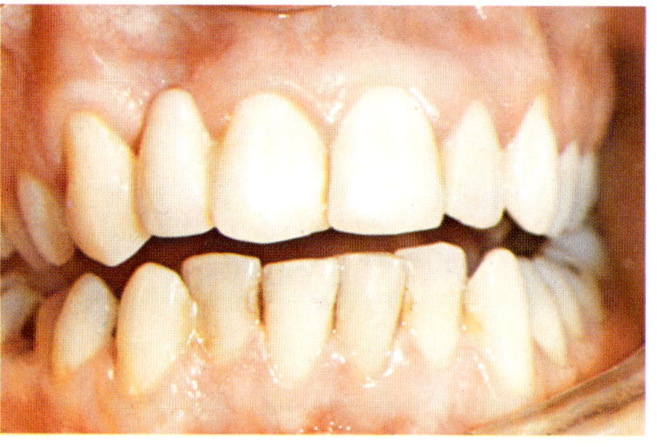

Fig. VI-16 Patient P. H. This anterior bridge was acid etched in place 30 months prior to this photograph. The maxillary right lateral incisor is an acrylic denture tooth which had retention for the Concise composite cut into the lingual. Many such bridges have lasted as long, but there is a weak link at the composite/pontic interface which will sooner or later break down.

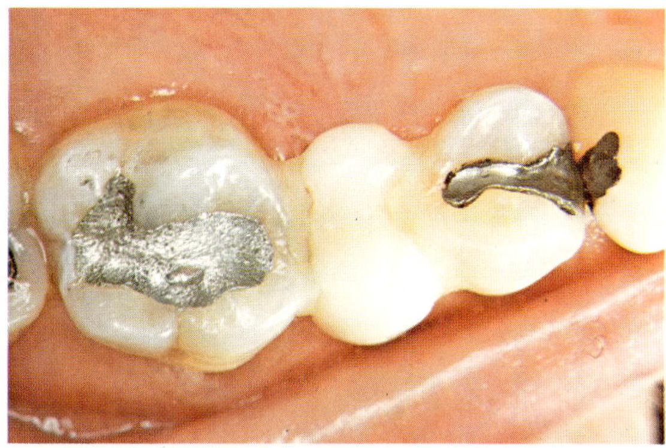

Fig. VI-17   Patient P. E. Posterior bridges can also be successfully placed utilizing the same technique. This patient had congenitally missing maxillary second bicuspids and wanted a simple, inexpensive replacement without going into gold preparations. A bicuspid denture tooth was trimmed down and locked into place with composite bonded to the adjacent teeth. This photograph is 28 months after placement.

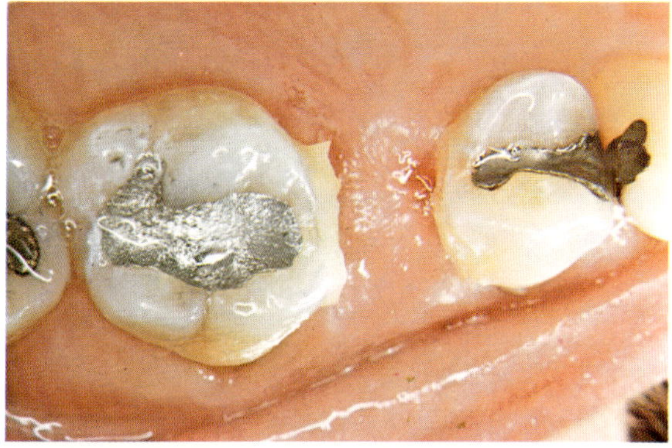

Fig. VI-18   Patient P. E. At 28 months after placement the denture tooth became loose as the composite/pontic interface broke down. The tooth was removed to again show how well the acid etch bond has been retained. It was decided to go into something somewhat more radical for added strength. The patient was extremely happy with the previous bridge and was very interested in trying the technique again.

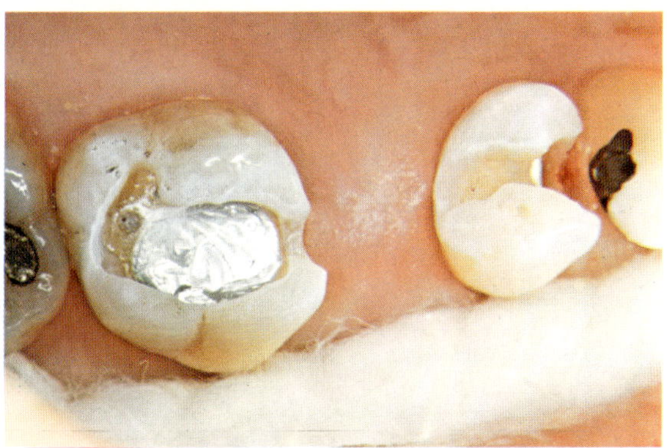

Fig. VI-19   Patient P. E. The old amalgams were removed from the abutment teeth except in the deepest areas. All margins were bevelled and the marginal ridges of the surface adjacent to the missing tooth removed enough so that a 0.81 mm wire could be added without interfering with occlusion. All enamel margins were etched after bases had been applied.

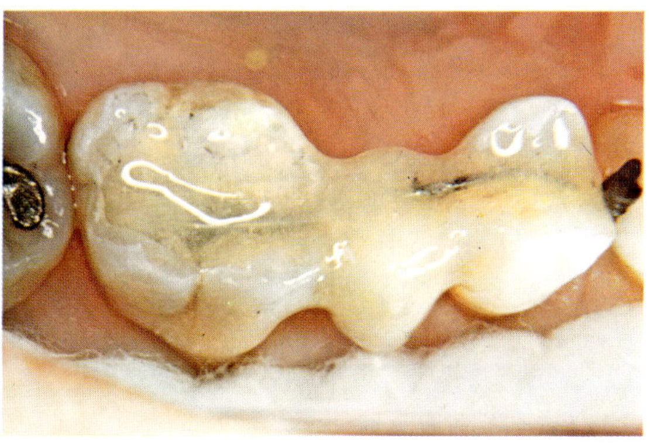

Fig. VI-20   Patient P. E. A wire was used to span the gap and give support to the composite pontic. All the preparations were filled with radiopaque composite (3M Concise experimental) and the complete bridge was glazed after grinding in the occlusion. The wire could have been placed deeper over the distal marginal ridge of the bicuspid, but minimal tooth preparation was a major consideration.

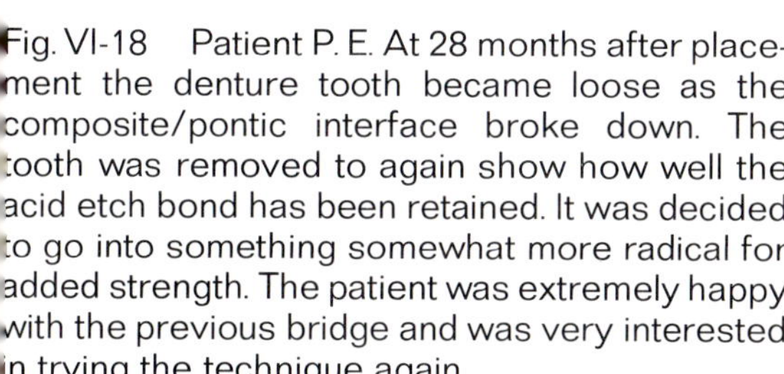

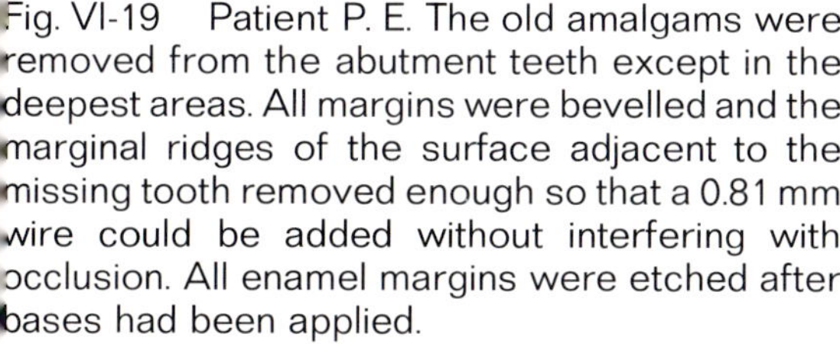

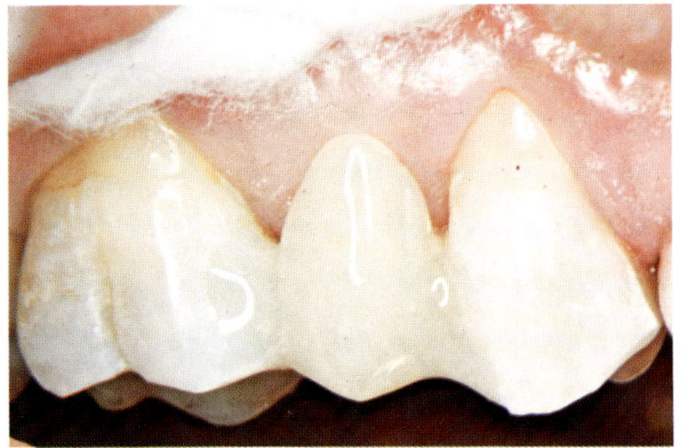

Fig. VI-21   Patient P. E. The finished bridge from the buccal aspect. The glaze can be seen to extend beyond the margins of composite on the abutment teeth. It is expected that bridges made in this manner will last longer than the 2–3 years one can expect from the use of acrylic denture teeth.

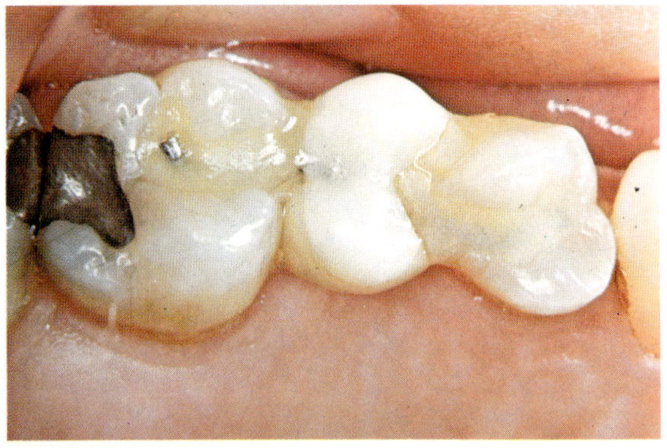

Fig. VI-22   Patient P. E. This bridge was placed on the opposite side of the mouth at the same time as Fig. VI-17 (28 months before photograph). A wire was used at that time for support and this has helped maintain the integrity of the composite/denture tooth interface. However, some breakdown of the anterior margin is already detectable.

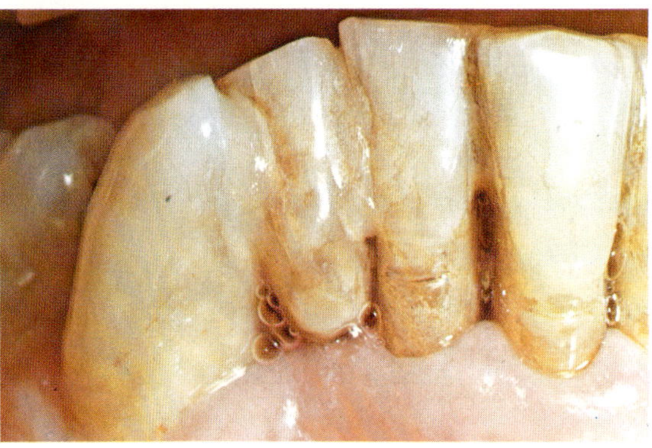

Fig. VI-23   Patient J. K. A different method of replacing a missing tooth is to use the patient's own tooth. This mandibular right lateral incisor was lost for periodontal reasons. The root was removed, the tooth adapted to the ridge and sealed apically with composite and glazed. After healing, the tooth was bonded into exactly the position it occupied previously. This photograph was taken at the 18 month recall appointment.

References

1. *Buonocore, M. G.:*
    The Use of Adhesives in Dentistry. Charles C. Thomas, Publisher, Springfield, Illinois, 1975.
2. *Ibsen, R. L. and Neville, K.:*
    Adhesive Restorative Dentistry, W. B. Saunders Co., Philadelphia, 1974.

    Joos, R. W.:
    Personal communication.
4. *Scheer, B. and Silverstone, L. M.:*
    Replacement of missing anterior teeth by etch retained bridges. J. Int. Ass. Dent. Child. 6: 17–19 1975.

Chapter 7

Acid Etched Class II Composite Restorations in the Deciduous Dentition

The silver amalgam has been the restorative material of choice for posterior restorations in dentistry, for many decades. The time is fast approaching, however, when the acid etched composite resin will be able to replace amalgam as the most-used dental restorative material, in adult, as well as pediatric, dentistry.

There is, at present, only one significant area where the composite is at a disadvantage as opposed to amalgam—namely wear. Present-day composites do not have the wear-characteristics of amalgam. Dental research in resin is, however, being directed towards the development of more wear-resistant composite systems. When such composite resins are available, the techniques described here for use in the deciduous dentition, will be applicable in the permanent dentition. The many other advantages of acid etched composites (particularly marginal integrity and a decrease in secondary decay) outweigh the wear disadvantage in deciduous teeth, which have a limited life-span. Thus, this author routinely uses acid etched composite for all deciduous restorations.

Advantages of acid etched composite resin compared to amalgam

1. Minimal tooth preparation—carious material only removed. No extension for prevention or mechanical retention preparation necessary.
2. The composite is bonded to all enamel margins. This reinforces the prepared tooth in a secondary manner. (Primarily, strength is gained by minimizing tooth preparation.)
3. The composite has much greater resistance to fracture. Particularly in pediatric dentistry, with large preparations in small teeth, amalgams have a tendency to fracture quite frequently.
4. Excellent marginal integrity. The acid etched margin is essentially leak-free and resistant to breakdown.
5. Improved esthetics. Although esthetics in the posterior of the mouth is not a big factor for children, when composites become recommended for adult dentistry, esthetics will be a major consideration.
6. No electrical or thermal conductivity. The seemingly inevitable period of sensitivity with newly-placed amalgam restorations, does not apply to composites.
7. Preventive restoration. The acid etch composite can be easily extended to sealing of remaining pits and fissures (technique explained in Chapter 8).
8. Smoother interproximal surfaces. It is almost impossible to polish an interproximal to a glaze smoothness, whether it be amalgam or composite, without losing contact. A properly placed

composite will require little interproximal attention, and the smoothness of composite placed against a Mylar strip is well known.

9. Occlusion can be checked immediately. As soon as the composite has polymerized, the patient can safely mark highspots with articulating paper, without fear of fracturing the restoration.
10. Polishing can be completed at the initial appointment. Amalgams must set for 24 hours prior to polishing. This means that the great majority of amalgams placed in general dentistry today, unfortunately do not get polished. Composites can be trimmed and polished immediately after polymerization is complete (approximately 4–5 minutes).

Disadvantages of acid etched composite resin compared to amalgam

1. Radiolucency. Initially, composites were radiolucent which meant that on x-ray they were indistinguishable from caries. However, both Johnson and Johnson (Adaptic) and 3M (Concise) now have excellent radiopaque composites (Fig. VII-20).
2. Wear. Undoubtedly this is the biggest drawback of resins when they are considered for use on the posterior teeth.
3. Technique. The skill necessary for successful acid etching requires a somewhat greater attention to the details of the technique.
4. Time. The placement of an acid etched composite takes 2–3 minutes longer than a similar amalgam restoration.

None of these disadvantages, except the wear factor, is significant for the operator concerned with placing the best possible restoration for his patients.

Technique

Minimal preparation is not only acceptable, but one of the major benefits of the technique. The only tooth structure removed is the carious material, or that enamel and dentin which must be removed in order to reach the carious lesion. No extension for prevention, or preparation for mechanical retention is necessary. After removal of carious material (Fig. VII-1), a small bevel is placed around all margins (Fig. VII-2), to remove loose enamel rods and improve the orientation of the prisms for etching.

After basing all dentin with calcium hydroxide base (Procal or Dycal), or with a liner (Zarosen), taking care not to contaminate any enamel margins, a matrix is placed. A Mylar strip cut into two lengthwise, and two across, makes four excellent and inexpensive matrices. Sometimes in the case of MOD restorations, it is better to use a metal matrix, such as the Caulk AutoMatrix seen in Figure VII-16. Proper wedging is essential for establishment of a good gingival margin and interproximal contact. Sometimes wedging from both buccal and lingual is desirable. Some separation of the teeth must be obtained by wedging, to obtain a good contact with the adjacent tooth.

When the matrix is complete, enamel margins are etched. (One need not be concerned with buccal and lingual margins not being flush with the matrix, since excess composite in these areas is easily trimmed down after polymerization with composite finishing burs.) In addition to etching enamel margins, the occlusal surface of the tooth being restored, and any occlusal pits and fissures on adjacent teeth, are etched. The etching time, with 37% phosphoric acid for deciduous enamel, presently recommended is 120 seconds. Sixty seconds is adequate when etching the occlusal surface only (Chapter 2), but the possible presence of "prismless" enamel, particularly in the cervical regions of the tooth, indicates that a 120-second etch is desirable for optimal etch pattern.

The etch is carried out as previously described. Throughout the etching time, the acid is continually replenished. After 2 minutes, the teeth etched are t h o r o u g h l y washed for at least 20 seconds for each tooth.

Enamel Bond resin is then applied to the dried, etched enamel with a disposable brush. A Centrix C-R syringe is loaded with 3M radiopaque Concise, and the composite is injected into the deepest portion of the cavity preparation first, filling the preparation from the inside to eliminate voids. The preparation is filled to excess and the Concise is flowed over the rest of the etched occlusal surface to:

1. Protect the rest of the pits and fissures from caries if necessary.
2. Utilize the etched enamel for retention.

Unfilled and filled resin (or a mix of White Sealant) is then applied to adjacent teeth also (Fig. VII-4), as necessary.

Polymerization takes place in about 4–5 minutes. The wedges and matrix are removed and the buccal and lingual excess trimmed down to the margins with a 7901 FG Midwest American carbide composite finishing bur.

The rubber dam is removed to check the occlusion. A 7408 FG Midwest American carbide bur is excellent for trimming down occlusal surfaces. The patient can bite down and give a clear bite registration with articulating paper, without fear of fracturing the restoration. A high spot, such as that seen in Figure VII-5, on the disto-marginal ridge of the freshly placed composite, should be removed.

Figure VII-6 shows the completed restoration with the heaviest contact on the enamel of the adjacent second deciduous molar. The White Sealant on the first permanent molar has been in place 12 months.

A further restorative series is seen in Figures VII-7 to 10. The DO in the first deciduous molar has been in place 12 months (Fig. VII-7). The restoration was in excellent condition. Caries was diagnosed on the mesial surface of the second molar. The tooth was prepared minimally, based with Zarosen liner, and completed as previously described.

Mesial caries can sometimes be successfully treated without involving the preparation of the marginal ridge. Figure VII-11 shows a mesial decalcification (soft) on the second deciduous molar exposed after preparing the DO in the first molar. The decalcification was scooped out with a round bur and the mesial surface etched and filled with Concise using a Mylar strip matrix. Where access permits, a re-etch and glaze application after polishing would be ideal. The first molar was then completed according to the technique previously described.

Figure VII-12 shows a mirror-view of the completed quadrant, with White Sealant on the occlusal of the second deciduous molar.

During routine restorative appointments, it is possible to extend the life of adjacent amalgams that are secondary-caries-free. The patient in Figure VII-13 has 5 or 6 separate amalgams in one occlusal surface! Rather than make the patient pay once again for treatment of the surface, the tooth can be sealed using the White Sealant resin mixed with some Concise catalyst paste (paste B), for added wear-resistance. The finished quadrant (Fig. VII-15), shows the full spectrum of resins from pure unfilled resin (White Sealant on the permanent molar), to a filled Concise resin restoration on the first deciduous molar, with a mix of both making a diluted filled resin on the second deciduous molar.

Resins in restorative dentistry are here to stay, as is the acid etch technique. The saving of tooth structure and greatly improved marginal integrity leading to a reduction in secondary caries, are major advantages when considering the use of acid etch composite resin restorations in the deciduous posterior dentition.

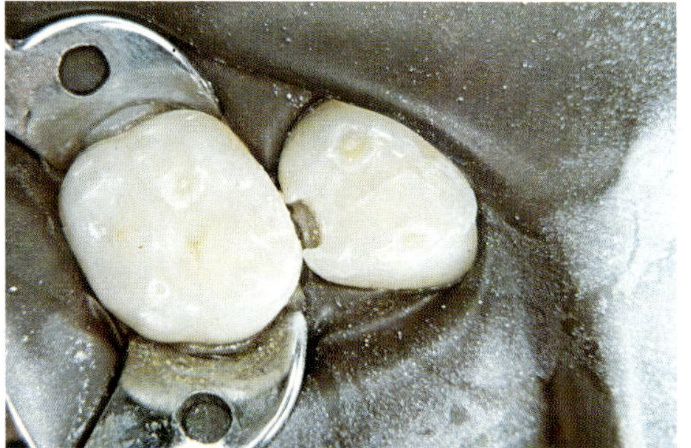

Fig. VII-1   Patient S.T. The radiopaque composite has many advantages over amalgam for deciduous restorative work. Use of composite allows minimal tooth preparation, it being necessary to remove only carious tooth structure or that which must be removed to reach carious enamel or dentin. No extension for prevention or extension into the occlusal surface is necessary, leaving a much stronger tooth.

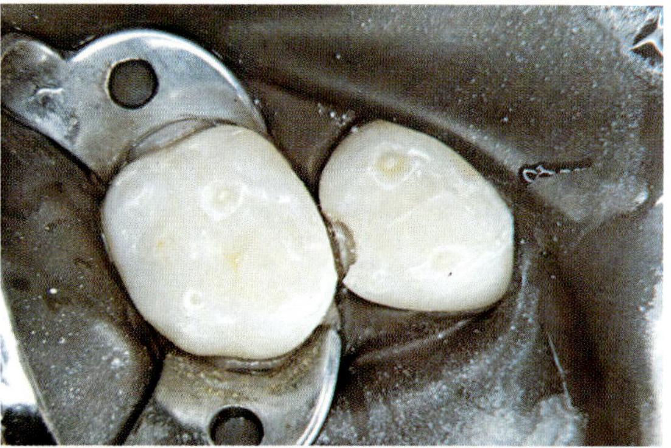

Fig. VII-2   Patient S.T. Minimal preparation is recommended since retention is gained from etching enamel margins and not from the cavity preparation. In this case the interproximal carious lesion has been removed and the enamel margins bevelled, including margins on the occlusal surface. Any exposed dentin is based with a calcium hydroxide base.

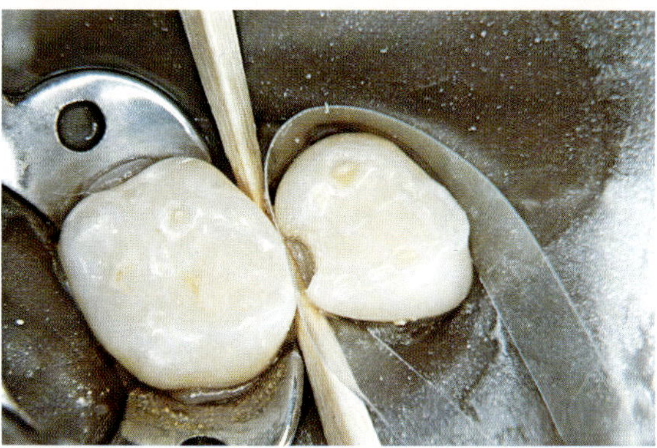

Fig. VII-3   Patient S.T. A Mylar strip cut into two lengthwise, and into two across, makes an excellent matrix. It is very thin and with adequate wedging for separation and gingival seat adaptation, there will be no problem with contact or with overhangs. Sometimes it is desirable to wedge from both buccal and lingual aspects to ensure an ideal gingival seat.

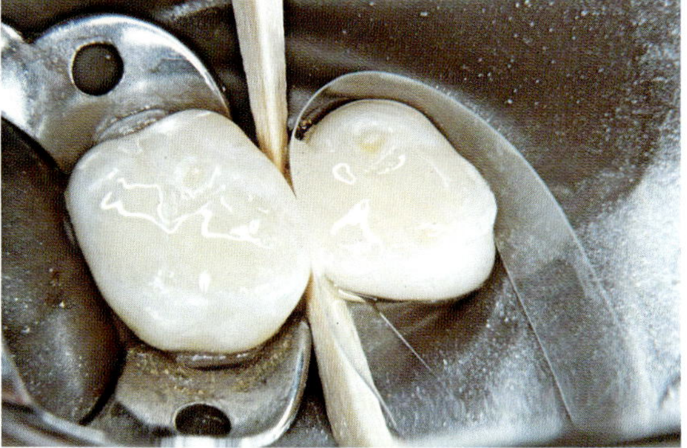

Fig. VII-4   Patient S.T. After etching, washing and drying (include the occlusal grooves of any other teeth isolated), the unfilled and then filled resin (3M Concise radiopaque experimental) was used. After polymerization the wedges and matrix are removed before trimming and polishing. The 7901 FG Midwest American carbide composite finishing bur is used initially to remove buccal and lingual excess (bur pictured Fig. V-5).

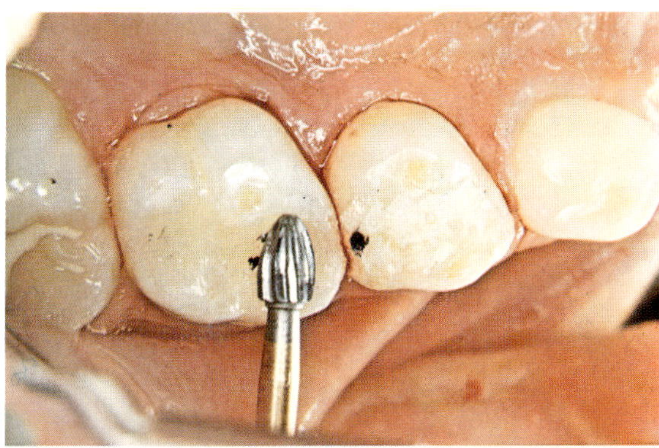

Fig. VII-5   Patient S. T. This composite finishing bur (7408 FG Midwest American carbide) is excellent for occlusal adjustment of composites. After removal of rubber dam, the occlusion should always be checked with articulating paper. Any high spots can then be taken down rapidly. It is an advantage of composite over amalgam that the occlusion can be thoroughly checked without fear of fracturing the restoration.

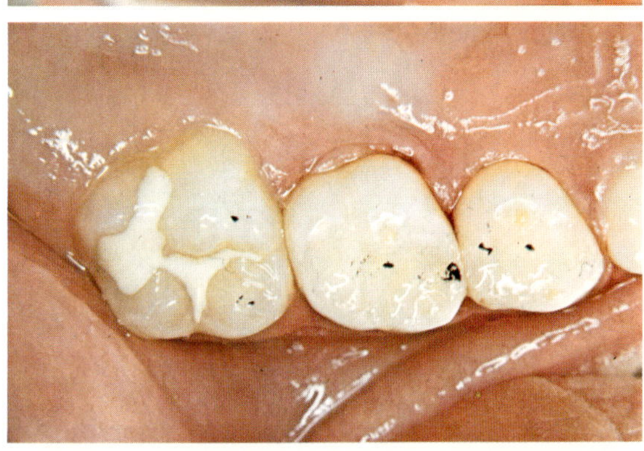

Fig. VII-6   Patient S.T. Once the occlusal contacts are light, or on enamel only, the restoration is complete. The glazing of these restorations is not usually routine, since addition of a glaze layer would only cover part of the restoration and the important area, the interproximal, is inaccessible to glaze. This area is, however, usually very smooth after placement with a Mylar strip.

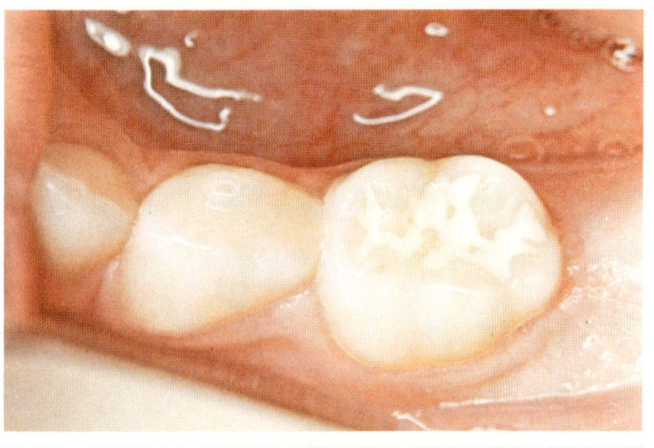

Fig. VII-7   Patient M. M. This DO restoration in the first deciduous molar has been in place 12 months, as has the occlusal sealant on the second molar. The restoration was in excellent condition with no marginal stain, breakdown or any significant amount of wear. At this time caries was diagnosed on the mesial of the second molar.

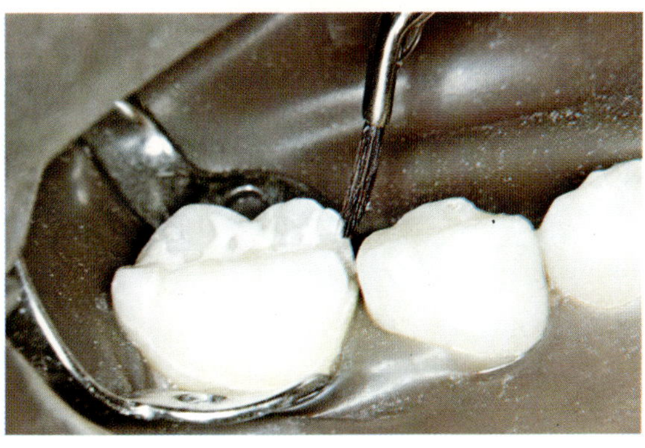

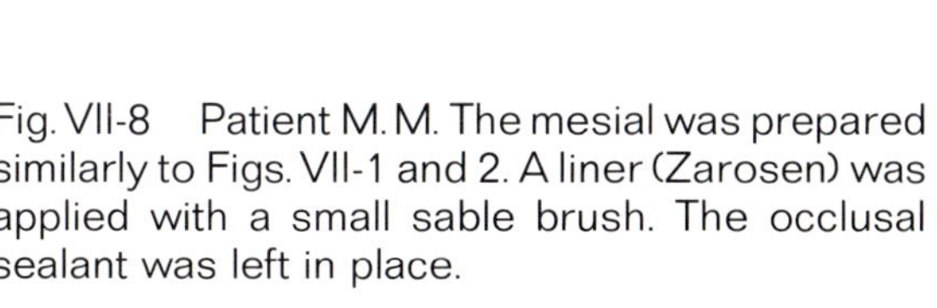

Fig. VII-8   Patient M. M. The mesial was prepared similarly to Figs. VII-1 and 2. A liner (Zarosen) was applied with a small sable brush. The occlusal sealant was left in place.

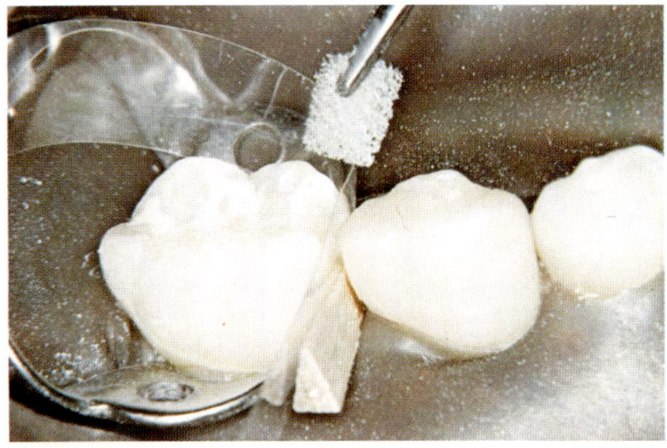

Fig. VII-9   Patient M. M. The bevelled enamel margins were etched for 120 seconds with 37% orthophosphoric acid using the 3M sponges for acid application.

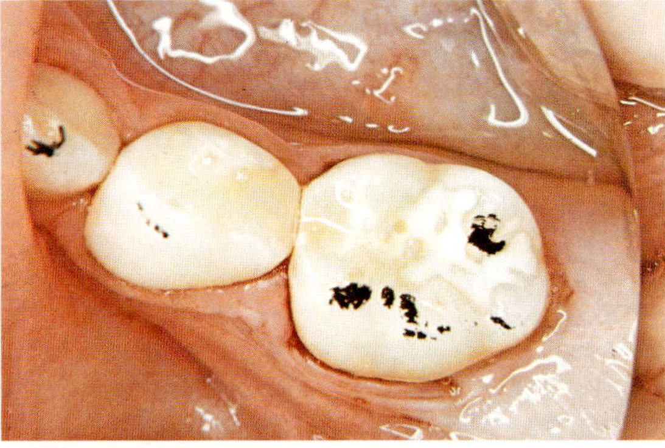

Fig. VII-10   Patient M. M. A mirror view of the finished restoration adjacent to the one year old DO in the first molar. The composite was simply merged into the sealant in the mesial marginal ridge area. The occlusion was checked to be sure no composite was causing an interference.

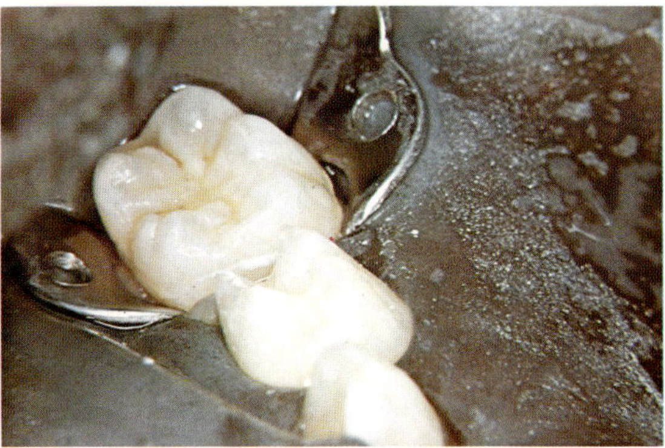

Fig. VII-11   Patient K. B. After preparing the DO in the first molar, the area of decalcification on the mesial of the second molar was found to be carious. This area was then scooped out while access was possible, without having to involve the marginal ridge in the preparation. The mesial was etched and restored with composite before the first molar was completed.

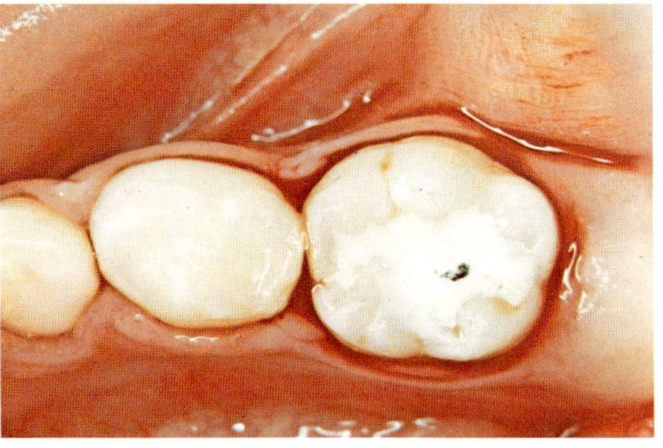

Fig. VII-12   Patient K. B. A mirror view of the finished DO in the first molar, with a sealant (3M White Sealant) placed on the occlusal of the second molar. The mesial on the second molar is of course not visible. Radiopaque composite is essential for such mesial spots. Amalgam or composite without acid etching is contraindicated in similar situations since marginal leakage inevitably leads to secondary caries attack.

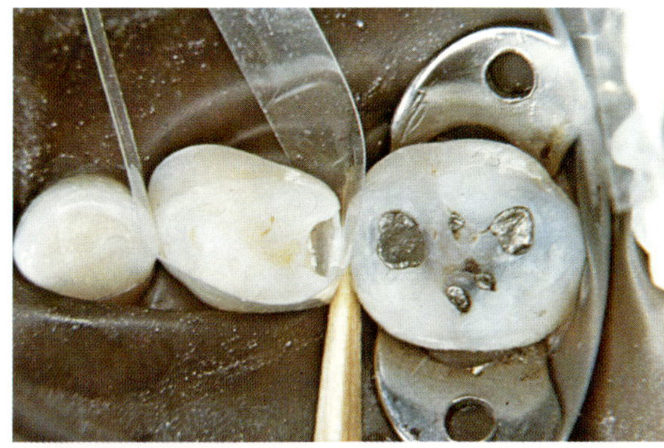

Fig. VII-13   Patient T. D. During routine restorative appointments it is frequently possible to extend the life of amalgams that as yet have no secondary caries. This patient has 5 (!) separate amalgams in the occlusal surface and it appears as if a sixth may have been lost. Rather than charge the patient for replacement, it is possible to seal over the amalgams, (pictured here after etching), to eliminate marginal leakage and consequent secondary decay.

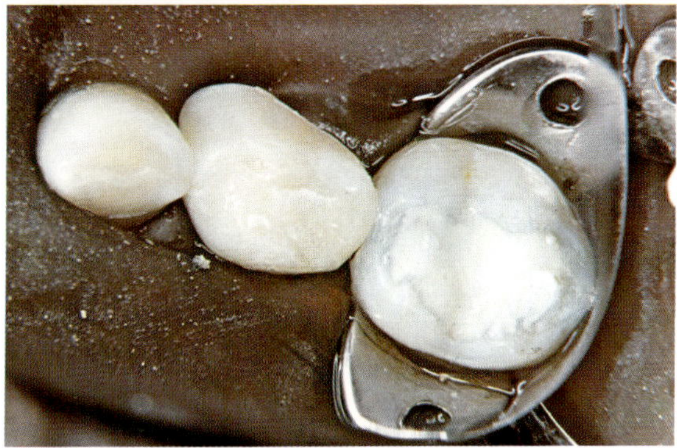

Fig. VII-14   Patient T. D. The DO in the first molar has been placed and the occlusal of the second molar sealed. In this case for added strength a diluted filled resin was used. The White resin A from the 3M White Sealant was mixed with Concise catalyst paste B. This gives, in effect, a filled sealant which will have more wear resistance, (desirable in this case), than the regular unfilled resin sealant.

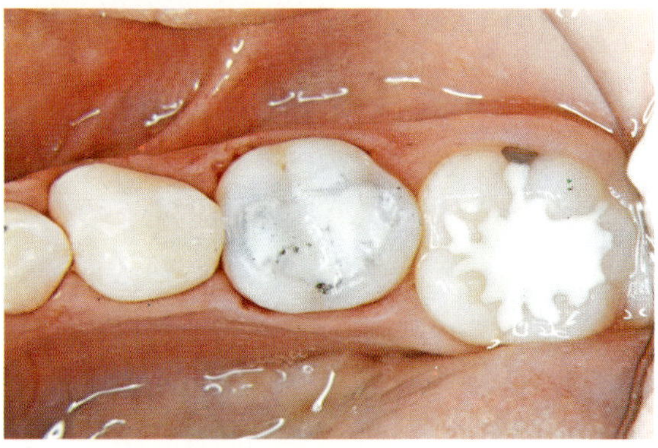

Fig. VII-15   Patient T. D. This patient shows in one quadrant the full spectrum of resin uses ranging from unfilled resin sealant on the first permanent molar, to a filled resin restoration on the first deciduous molar, with a mix of both making a diluted filled resin, (or filled sealant), on the second deciduous molar.

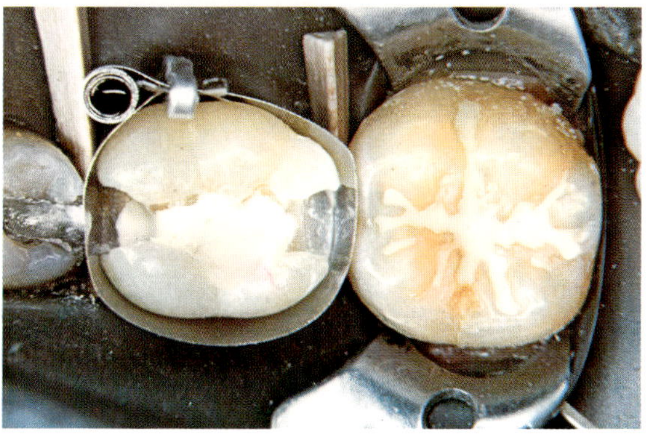

Fig. VII-16   Patient T. E. For MOD restorations it is sometimes better to use a conventional amalgam matrix such as this thin Caulk AutoMatrix. Proper wedging will still enable adequate contact to be obtained.

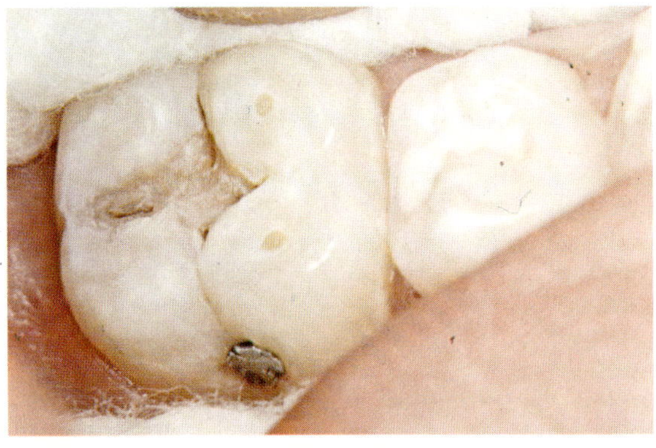

Fig. VII-17   Patient J. D. This first permanent molar has lost an occlusal amalgam. The tooth was caries-free and was etched for composite placement.

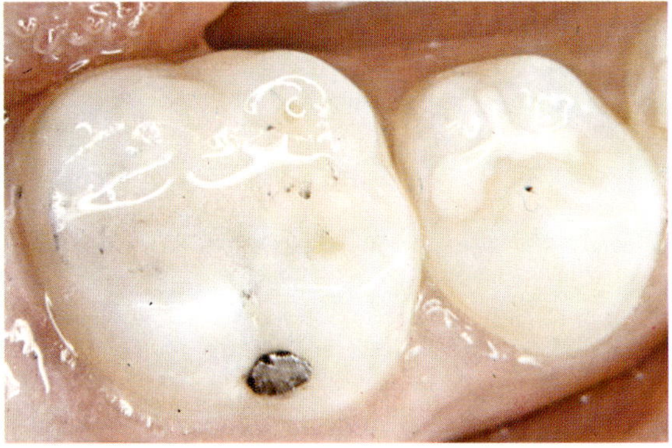

Fig. VII-18   Patient J. D. 3M Concise was bonded to the occlusal surface. Although composites will wear down more rapidly than amalgams, future research will undoubtedly be in the direction of more wear-resistant composites, so that their use in the permanent dentition can be expanded to include multi-surface lesions.

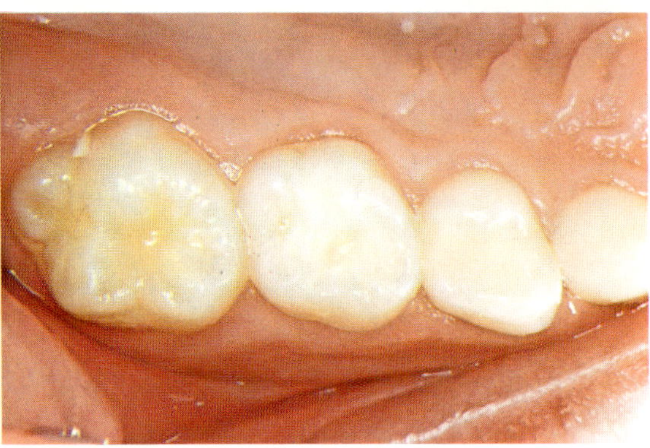

Fig. VII-19   Patient K. S. This patient has a DO in the first deciduous molar that was placed 15 months before this photograph. The diluted Concise sealant (Chapter VIII) is 20 months old and after further eruption of the tooth some White Sealant was added to a newly exposed portion of the groove that was not previously covered.

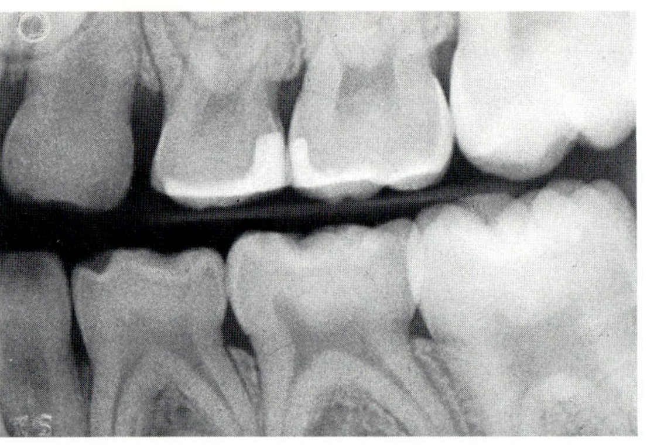

Fig. VII-20   Patient S. T. An x-ray taken at 12 month recall of two adjacent 3M Concise experimental radiopaque composite restorations. The radiopacity is not equal to that of amalgam, but it is sufficient that even a thin occlusal layer can be detected when viewed from the buccal on a bitewing x-ray.

Chapter 8

Preventive Resin Restorations

A technique for caries restoration and simultaneous caries prevention had been an impossible dream before the introduction of the acid etch technique. Now it is possible to lay aside the old techniques of the prophylactic odontotomy, of fissure eradication and of extension for prevention. It is now not only possible, but recommended, to use composites and the acid etch system, to restore carious lesions and prevent secondary caries concurrently.

The prophylactic odontotomy was born in 1923 with *Hyatt's*[8] publication of a paper dealing with the restoration of potentially carious pits and fissures. The prophylactic odontotomy is in use even now, 55 years later. The technique undoubtedly has served the purpose of reducing the size of the preparation necessary by restoring potentially carious areas prior to caries attack taking hold. Just as certainly, however, some teeth that never would have decayed were subjected to a restorative procedure.

Smoothing the cuspal slopes to flatten out the sharp pits and fissures, thus making them easier to keep clean, rather than restoring them, was another frequently used method of caries prevention.[2] This technique also is still in use today, although rarely. The improvement in, and increasing use of, pit and fissure sealants and composite resins has rendered these techniques obsolescent.

After diagnosis of caries in pits and fissures, amalgam is presently accepted by most practitioners as the restorative material of choice. Many questionably carious or "sticky" fissures are restored with amalgam. Several problems relating to the use of amalgam for single surface restorations have propelled composite resins, used with the acid etch technique, to the forefront of clinical dental research. Over-preparation (Fig. VIII-1), marginal leakage, marginal breakdown and secondary caries are all problems of amalgam restorations in young permanent molars. Frequently, these problems lead to severe weakening of the tooth structure, sometimes in just a few years post-eruption. Many of these teeth become destined for full gold crowns, as much from weaknesses in preparation technique and material properties, as from the primary caries attack.

It has always been this author's goal to seek out the most conservative approach possible to any restorative procedure. If this approach fails, it is then always possible to go one step further with a more radical technique. Thus, the old and still much-used adage of "extension for prevention" sometimes brought serious doubts to mind when an occlusal surface riddled with supplemental grooves, and having just one small spot of caries, was observed (Fig. VIII-2). What does one do? Is it best to restore each area as decay is diagnosed, (and have the tooth look like it received a shot–gun blast, Fig. VII-13, as well as having the patient pay for one surface several times more than is necessary), or does one remove all the occlusal anatomy and severely weaken the tooth? (Fig. VIII-1.) Fortunately, one does not often have to make such a decision and "extension for prevention" can still result in some very conservative restorations that snake their way over the occlusal surface. Inevitably, however, healthy tooth substance is removed in order to prevent decay from attacking at another site on the same tooth (this is an extension of *Hyatt's* principle).

The challenge, then, is to restore minimal carious lesions (usually in young permanent teeth) with the minimum of tooth removal, and at the same time, prevent caries from attacking other pits and fissures on the same surface. To this end, this author has been using a technique which he calls preventive resin restoration. This technique uses a scale to judge cavity size and thus pick the filled/unfilled resin combination suitable for use. At the time of writing, patients have been seen that were treated in a study initiated two years ago. The results are so promising that this technique, or some similar one utilizing composite resin, may well replace the silver amalgam as the restorative material of choice for minimal single surface restorations in posterior teeth in the near future. With further improvement in the wear-characteristics of the composite resin, routine use of the material for multiple surface restorations is foreseen.

Earlier, problems relating to the use of amalgam in restoring pit and fissure caries, were alluded to.

These problems are:

1. Extension for prevention removes much healthy tooth structure. Over-preparation weakens the tooth more than necessary.

2. Secondary caries can attack the margins of the amalgam restoration quite rapidly, particularly in areas of supplemental grooves adjacent to an amalgam margin. Fissures not included in the preparation are also susceptible to attack.
3. Marginal leakage: all amalgam restorations exhibit some degree of marginal leakage, which can lead to secondary caries.
4. Marginal breakdown: all amalgam restorations, particularly those on occlusal surfaces that contain a lot of supplemental anatomy, are subject to marginal breakdown. Unpolished restorations particularly exhibit rapid marginal breakdown.
5. For some people, esthetics are important, even in the posterior teeth, and amalgam is not an esthetically acceptable material.

All of these problems are overcome when using unfilled and/or filled composite resins for the preventive resin restoration (PRR) that is to be described here. In any event, should the PRR fail, amalgam can always be used later. It is not possible to make a PRR from a failed amalgam.

Indications for Preventive Resin Restorations:

1. Explorer "catch" in a pit or fissure.
2. Minimal pit and fissure caries.
3. Deep pits and fissures with much supplemental anatomy and small areas of decay.

Contraindication for Preventive Resin Restorations:

1. Large single- or multi-surface carious lesions.

Advantages of Preventive Resin Restorations:

1. Less tooth structure is removed, leaving

a much stronger tooth than when extension for prevention is necessary.
2. Eliminates marginal leakage and secondary decay.
3. Prevents decay in adjacent pits and fissures without fissure removal. .
4. Patient suffers less discomfort from mechanical tooth removal (anesthesia is seldom needed for PRR).
5. Patient does not need to be rescheduled for polishing (as for amalgam restorations).
6. PRR can be easily added to, or replaced, without further tooth preparation.

Disadvantages of Preventive Resin Restorations:

1. Require strict attention to detail and absolute adherence to the principles of acid etching.
2. The procedure takes possibly 2–3 minutes per tooth longer than a single-surface amalgam restoration.
3. The long-term retention and wear, compared to well-placed amalgams, has yet to be determined.

Research Background:

Preliminary in vitro studies were undertaken at the University of Minnesota (*Simonsen* 1973 unpublished) prior to clinical application of the technique. In vitro studies show that the dilution of 3M Concise with Enamel Bond unfilled resin in various ratios resulted in a mix that invariably handled much more easily than the pure, filled or unfilled, resin.
After completion of the in vitro studies, a clinical study to test the PRR was initiated at Group Health Medical Center in Bloomington, Minnesota. Children were selected for the study who exhibited minimal carious areas or questionable "sticky" fissures.
The preventive dental health program at Group Health Medical Center consists of bite wing and panographic radiography, oral hygiene instructions, pumice prophylaxis, topical fluoride treatment and sealant treatment, as necessary. After examination of radiographs for any sign of interproximal or occlusal caries, the occlusal surfaces were thoroughly examined using a sharp no. 5 Star-Lite explorer. The occlusal surfaces were graded according to *Hinding* and *Buonocore*[7].

0. Surface free of explorer "catch" and the enamel translucent and continuous.
1. Explorer "catch" in fissure or pit but no resistance to explorer removal; enamel translucent with no color changes.
2. Explorer "catch" under moderate pressure; stickiness and resistance to removal evident but no opaque areas or softness; the adjacent area firm.
3. (Carious); discontinuity of enamel caused by loss of tooth substance; or a "catch" was evident and an opaque area adjacent to the pit and fissure; softness at the base of the area or loss of normal enamel translucency was present.

In deciding whether to use only unfilled resin or a combination of unfilled and filled resin, the graded teeth were split into groups.

Group A: Consists of teeth in occlusal grade 0 and 1. All teeth in this group, even those requiring a minimal exploratory preparation, were sealed with 3M Concise Brand White Sealant System.

Group B: Consists of teeth in occlusal grade 2. All teeth in this group were subject to some form of exploratory preparation with a round bur. If no caries was found, the White Sealant was used. If caries was found, the preparation was enlarged until all caries had been removed and the tooth was sealed/restored with dilute Concise placed on top of an intermediate unfilled resin layer.

Group C: Consists of teeth in occlusal grade 3. Minimal preparations were sealed/restored with dilute Concise, while those that became large enough for the introduction of a composite syringe were usually treated with a pure unfilled intermediate resin, then pure filled resin.

Technique

The PRR gradation of Groups A, B and C were treated as follows:

Group A: All teeth were sealed as previously described in Chapter 2. These teeth were usually treated at the same time other teeth were receiving sealant, thus cotton roll isolation was considered adequate for the reasons previously described (Chapter 2). No base or liner was used.

Group B: After exploration of the explorer "catch" with as small a round bur as possible, it was decided whether the tooth could be treated as in Group A, or if a dilute Concise PRR was indicated. If caries was found, necessitating further exploration until an area of sound dentin was reached, a dilute Concise restoration was indicated. Using some filled resin in the unfilled resin adds strength and abrasion resistance that is necessary at the cavo-surface margin (Figs. VIII-2 to 7). Sometimes, on lower molars where only the buccal pit was involved, dilute Concise was used on the buccal surface and White Sealant on the occlusal surface (Figs. VIII-8 to 10). If there were two or more areas prepared, or if it was desired to expedite the technique, dilute Concise was used over all remaining pits and fissures after restoring the preparation (Fig. VIII-12).

Many teeth treated with dilute Concise have been successfully treated using cotton roll isolation. At the present time, there appears to be no significant difference in retention for those treated with cotton roll isolation and those treated under rubber dam. In most cases, however, there is no doubt that use of the rubber dam is indicated to ensure a dry field and to retract the gingiva from an otherwise inaccessible subgingival groove (such as the lingual of upper molars or buccal of lower molars).

A very small round bur "size 0" is used initially to remove the questionable pit or fissure. Very careful clinical examination is necessary at this time to ensure that all caries has been removed. A stained pit need not be completely removed unless softness is detected with an explorer. The dilute Concise is then prepared while the tooth is being etched for 60 seconds with 37% orthophosphoric acid, using a small sponge held in a self-locking cotton plier. Care must be taken to etch at least 2 mm beyond the margin of the exploratory preparation, as well as over all other exposed pits and fissures (Fig. VIII-6).

The mixture chosen for dilute Concise, was one drop of universal resin (resin A) to an approximately equal amount of universal paste (paste A) and one drop of catalyst resin (resin B) to an equal amount of catalyst paste (paste B). Slightly more catalyst than universal paste is used to increase the setting and working time. These two mixes are held apart until needed, and then mixed together. The resultant dilute Concise was found to be easily picked up with any instrument. Various instruments for application were tried before deciding that a regular explorer (Star-Lite no. 5) is most suitable for two reasons:

1. It is invariably present on any restorative set-up. Using one instrument for more than one use cuts down on the complexity and cost of tray set-ups.
2. The instrument is finely pointed enough to introduce the material to the very smallest preparation.

The dilute Concise, when mixed as described, flows very freely over an etched surface. Care must be taken not to trap air in very small preparations. Using the explorer carefully and allowing the material to run down one wall of the preparation until the cavity is filled from the inside, ensures wetting the cavity walls.

The use of a pure unfilled intermediate resin layer has caused some dispute in the literature as to its necessity. Some authors, such as *Dreyer Jorgensen,*[5] *Raadal*[10] and *Asmussen,*[1] feel that equal "tag" length can be obtained with the use of filled or unfilled resins on etched enamel. *Asmussen* showed "tags" of 50 microns with both unfilled and filled resins. Authors such as *Silverstone,*[14] however, have reported "tags" of 100 microns from unfilled resin. It is extremely difficult to prepare specimens of unfilled resin "tags", as the tags are extremely friable and almost any preparation technique will fracture the longest tags, leaving a layer of "base tags". These "base tags" may well appear to be as long with filled or unfilled resin, but that does not discount unfilled resin producing longer "tags".

An important question yet to be answered is, if tags of equal length are obtained, such as some authors claim, are the tags of equal density and do they fill in voids created by etching as well as unfilled resins? Authors such as *Buonocore*[3] and *Mohammed, Schoen* and *Burrell*[9] showed superior bond strength when an intermediate resin layer is used. *Dogon,*[4] *Buonocore*[3] and *Forsten*[6] have shown that microleakage is virtually eliminated when an intermediate resin layer is used, whereas pure filled resin on etched enamel exhibits considerable leakage.

In a recent (1977) personal communication, *Raadal*[11] reports that pure filled resin gives a stronger bond than diluted resin (both applied on etched enamel without use of an intermediate resin layer). *Magne Raadal* and his Norwegian colleague, *Harald Ulvestad* have both been working for several years with composite resins and have completed some excellent studies.

The first preventive sealant restorations placed by this author, were without the intermediate unfilled resin layer. However, the step of placing the unfilled resin onto the etched enamel before the diluted composite was soon adopted, as it was felt at the time, that better "tag" formation (and thus better retention) along with less microleakage would result. (It was also easier to introduce the dilute Concise into small preparations without trapping air, if a dilute resin was already present.) The application of the intermediate resin layer does not significantly lengthen the time of the procedure and, since it probably is helpful, and certainly does no harm, there is no reason to omit it. *Forsten's*[6] study has confirmed the benefit of the intermediate resin layer, concluding, "The results indicate the advantage of using an intermediary resin with etching even when the composite is diluted."

It is desirable in most Group B cases, to protect exposed dentinal tubules with some form of base. It is very difficult to introduce a calcium hydroxide base, such as Dycal or Procal, into a small preparation using the usual applicating instrument, as most of the base ends up on the walls of the preparation rather than the floor. Similarly, liners on cotton pellets would cover a lot of enamel externally and this may hinder etching. So, despite the fact that Zinc Oxide and Eugenol is supposed to hinder curing of resin in contact with it, it has been used successfully as a base with no apparent ill-effects. The ZOE is mixed very thickly and some Zinc Acetate is added to speed the setting. Then a very small amount is rolled up into a ball and carried to the preparation on as large an amalgam plugger as will fit into the preparation, or on a cut-off explorer tip (Fig. VIII-11). This ZOE is easily condensed onto the floor of the preparation with no contamination of enamel walls and it sets rapidly. Once set, it is not thought that the Eugenol will hinder the composite cure, and even if it did, it would be of no consequence to the final strength of the PRR, as it would be below the area of etch retained resin. After basing and etching, an unfilled resin layer is applied, using a disposable brush. While the unfilled resin is being applied, the assistant is mixing the two diluted portions of universal and catalyst resins, (A and B), which are then applied immediately, using the explorer as described. All remaining pits and fissures in the tooth are covered to the same degree that they would be covered with White Sealant.

Figure VIII-12 shows a deciduous second molar with dilute Concise applied. Lately, the White Sealant has been incorporated into the dilute Concise. Using one drop of the White Resin A and mixing it with an equal amount of the catalyst paste B from the Concise orthodontic resin kit, (the Concise here containing 6% less filler), one gets a mix of similar consistency to dilute Concise. Using this mix eliminates the step of diluting the pastes A and B with resins A and B prior to the final mix, as was previously used for dilute Concise preventive resin restorations. White dilute Concise is seen in Figures VIII-4 and 7.

Group C: Almost invariably rubber dam and local anesthesia are desirable for treating teeth in this group. Extra heavy rubber dam and Ivory no. 14 retainer are ideal for most permanent molars. Deciduous molars would require a W8A retainer, whereas partially erupted permanent molars need a no. 14A retainer, which retracts the gingiva very well.

Caries removal is accomplished using the smallest round bur that is just large enough to remove fresh enamel at all margins, (usually size no. 1 or no. 2 round bur for this type of lesion). Great care must be taken to check for lateral dentinal spread of caries along the dentino-enamel junction. If in doubt, the enamel margins are extended.

Basing these preparations that extend into dentin is absolutely necessary, as all composite resins cause temporary inflammatory responses in the pulp. Although it is felt that these reactions are reversible (also those from H_3PO_4) if the dentin has at least a thickness of 1 mm, there is no reason to take a chance on a pulpal reaction when bases can be easily applied.

If the preparation is small, the technique for basing and sealing/restoring as described for Group B can be followed. If the preparation is large enough for a calcium hydroxide base instrument, with a drop of Dycal or Procal, to be introduced, this should be done. The tooth should then be etched (Fig. VIII-19) and unfilled resin applied as before. Immediately after this, pure filled resin can be mixed and applied, utilizing a Centrix C-R syringe (Fig. VIII-20). This resin can also be carried, (although with slightly more difficulty than the dilute Concise), over the unfilled resin layer covering other exposed pits and fissures, thus sealing these areas with a filled resin. Such restorations should always be checked after rubber dam removal and before the patient is dismissed, to be sure that they are not causing an occlusal interference. Pure unfilled resin is of no concern if causing an initial occlusal interference. The resin will wear down in a day or two of occlusal abrasion. As more filled resin is added, however, it takes longer to wear down the interference. Therefore, occlusal adjustment should be routine for filled resin preventive restorations.

Study Results

Harald Ulvestad,[15–17] a pioneer in the use of dilute Concise as a fissure sealant, has reported excellent results from his studies. The technique differs somewhat from the dilute Concise technique described previously in this chapter. *Ulvestad* shares the view of *Dreyer Jorgensen*[5], *Raadal*[10] and *Asmussen*[1], maintaining that the penetration of resin tags with filled or unfilled resin into etched enamel is comparable. *Ulvestad*[18] feels very strongly that the intermediate resin layer, as favored by most researchers in the United States, is of no value. *Dogon*[4], *Buonocore*[3] and others disagree with *Ulvestad* and his Scandinavian colleagues. Looking objectively at studies available, this author feels more comfortable using the intermediate resin layer than omitting it. The evidence of decreased microleakage and increased bond strength means more than studies which show equal tag lengths from filled or unfilled resins. The question of tag density and amount of enamel prism volume filled has not been addressed by the "no-intermediate-resin-layer-group". Studies such as those of *Raadal*[11] and *Dreyer Jorgensen*[5] prove that short tags can be obtained with both filled and unfilled resin. They do not prove that long tags can be found with a filled resin (such as tags in excess of 50–90 microns).

Ulvestad's[17] three-year publication reported 92% retention in occlusal surfaces using dilute Concise and 67% retention using Nuva-Seal using both materials purely as pit and fissure sealants (no tooth preparation). The retention in buccal fissures is reported to be 91% for dilute Concise versus 74% with Nuva-Seal. *Simonsen*[13] reported 100% retention in lingual and buccal fissures, as well as in occlusal surfaces, after 12 months, using dilute Concise as a preventive resin restoration. After 24 months, there has not been any breakdown or loss of the cases seen at 12 months. Some teeth required additional dilute Concise or White Sealant, as previously unerupted grooves either became carious or became susceptible to decay by erupting further (Fig. VII-19 and Fig. VIII-17). At 24 months, wear of the dilute Concise becomes a factor. Fig. VIII-13 shows a 24-month occlusal and buccal dilute Concise. Wear was greatest at the occlusal portion of the buccal groove and this area will soon require additional material (pure filled resin may be better) as the diluted resin wears below the level of the cavity walls.

The technique of utilizing diluted filled composite resins has been shown to be an effective method of pit and fissure sealing (*Ulvestad*[15,16,17]). The further application of the technique to restoring minimal carious lesions concurrently with sealing the remaining pits and fissures, described in this chapter and called preventive resin restoration, has been shown to be clinically effective. It is hoped the technique will be used by more clinicians to save unnecessary removal of healthy tooth structure and to eliminate further tooth destruction from secondary caries.

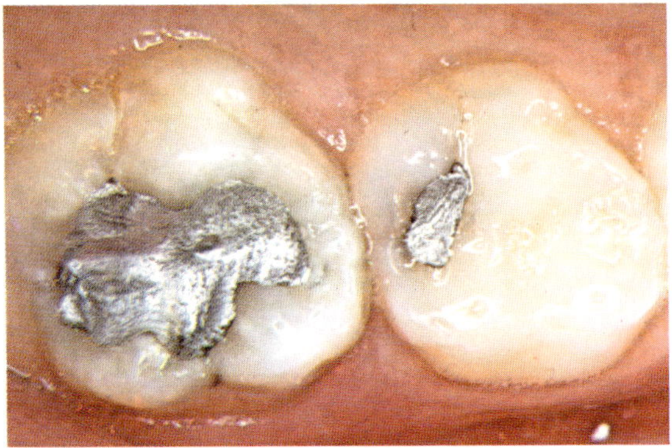

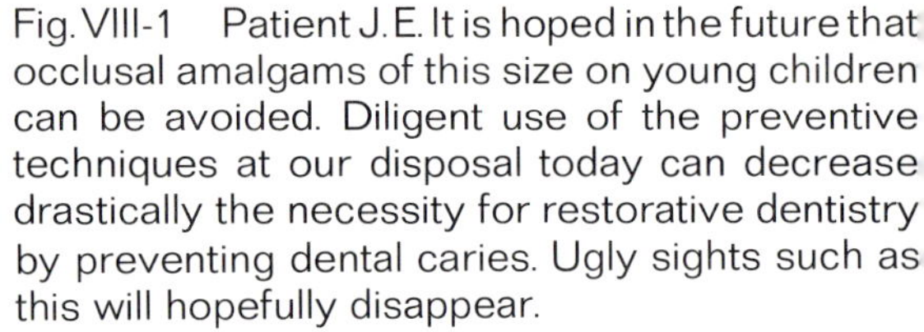

Fig. VIII-1   Patient J. E. It is hoped in the future that occlusal amalgams of this size on young children can be avoided. Diligent use of the preventive techniques at our disposal today can decrease drastically the necessity for restorative dentistry by preventing dental caries. Ugly sights such as this will hopefully disappear.

Fig. VIII-2   Patient P. F. In the past, small lingual lesions such as on this first permanent molar would be incorporated into an occluso-lingual preparation for amalgam, according to the extension-for-prevention philosophy. This type of preparation, however, necessarily removes a lot of healthy tooth structure. The acid etch technique enables one to prevent decay without removing healthy tooth structure.

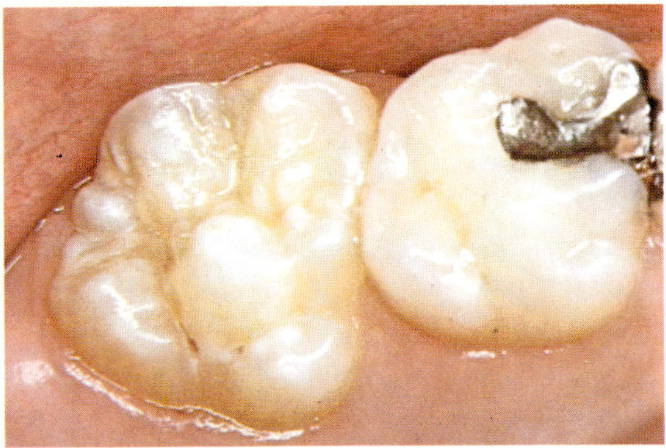

Fig. VIII-3   Patient P. F. The size of the preparation necessary for caries removal determines what will be used to seal/restore the tooth. In this case the preparation is so small that pure unfilled resin (White Sealant) could be used. However, since the preparation is on a surface exposed to wear, it was decided to add some filled resin for increased strength.

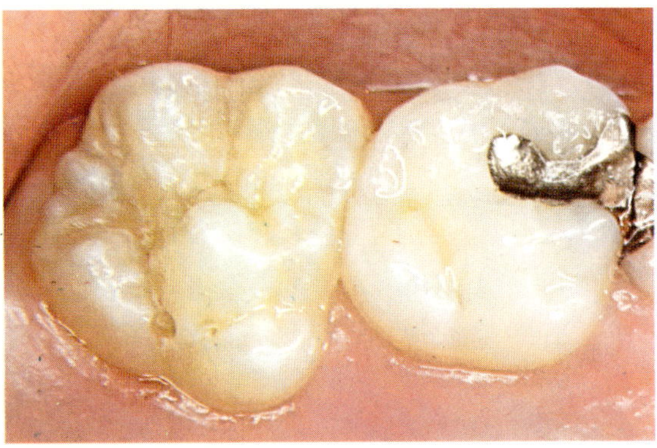

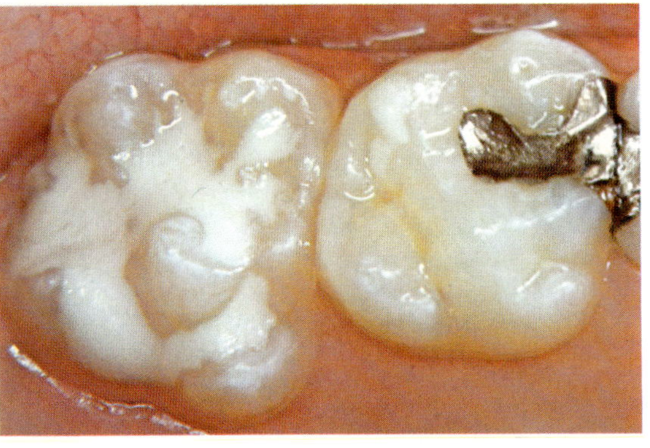

Fig. VIII-4   Patient P. F. The filled sealant has a rougher surface than the pure White Sealant as some filler particles are on the surface. A layer of pure unfilled resin (Enamel Bond) is always added under any mixture of filled resin and unfilled resin. When filled resin is added, the occlusion should always be checked upon completion, and high spots removed.

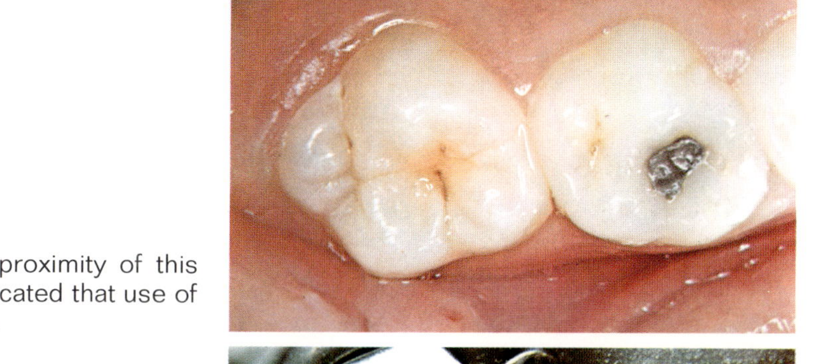

Fig. VIII-5   Patient T. D. The proximity of this lingual lesion to the gingiva indicated that use of the rubber dam was necessary.

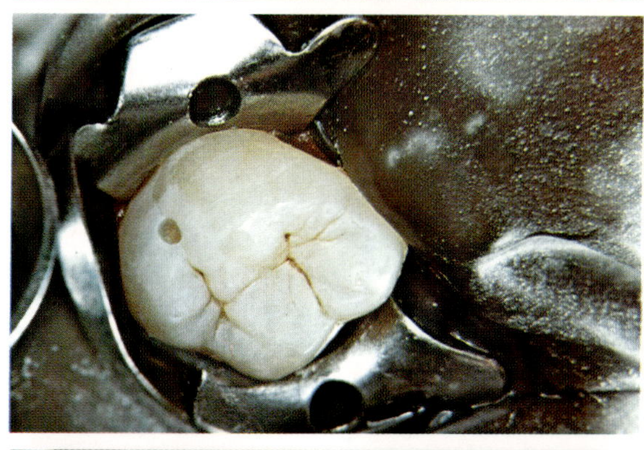

Fig. VIII-6   Patient T. D. After removing all the caries the tooth was etched for 60 seconds with 37% orthophosphoric acid. The etch should be carried about 2 mm beyond the margins of the preparation to be sure that there will be no leakage around the margins. The size and location of this preparation indicated that some addition of filled resin would be beneficial.

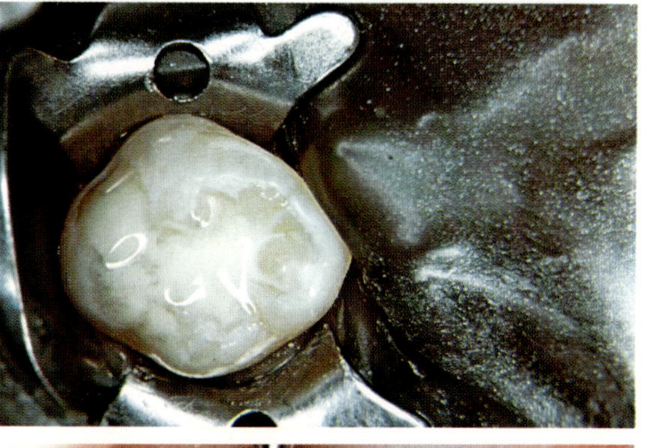

Fig. VIII-7   Patient T. D. Mixing Concise catalyst resin with the White Sealant (resin A) forms a filled sealant ideal for sealant-restorations. A layer of pure unfilled resin (Enamel Bond) is applied to assure plentiful unfilled resin for "tag" formation. There is disagreement in the literature on the necessity for this step (see text on page 93). Occlusion should be checked after removal of the rubber dam.

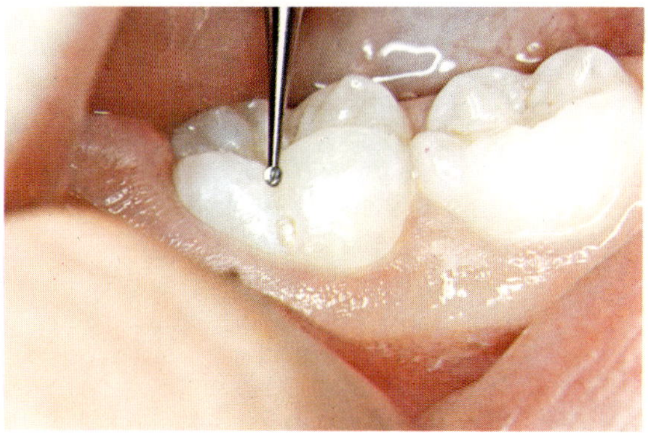

Fig. VIII-8   Patient J. J. Buccal lesions of this kind are seen frequently soon after eruption of mandibular first permanent molars. The soft material should be removed with a small round bur making the preparation as small as possible. A base should be applied if dentin is exposed.

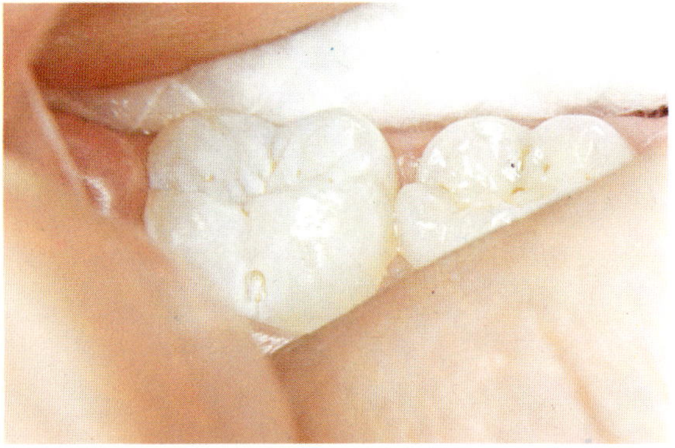

Fig. VIII-9   Patient J. J. This case was completed using cotton roll isolation. The tooth has now been etched, the etch being carried beyond the wall of the preparation by about 2 mm. It was decided in this case to use White Sealant on the occlusal and dilute Concise on the buccal for added strength and wear resistance in the cavity preparation.

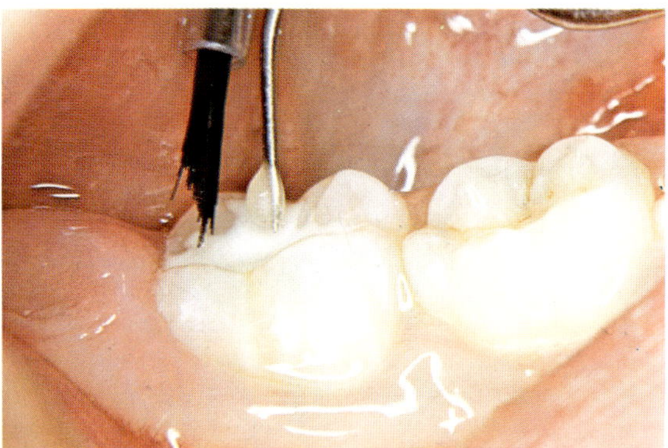

Fig. VIII-10   Patient J. J. Dilute Concise is best applied using an explorer tip which picks the material up nicely. An unfilled resin layer is applied first which aids in flow of the dilute Concise. White Sealant was applied to the occlusal surface using a disposable brush, although in most cases where dilute Concise is used on any part of the tooth it is used over all the pits and fissures.

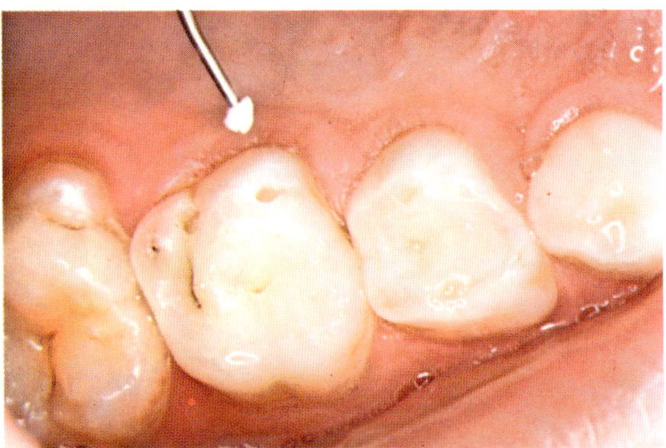

Fig. VIII-11   Patient C. M. Some very small preparations become quite deep. It is difficult to introduce calcium hydroxide without getting the base all down the walls of the preparation, and none at the floor. Zinc oxide and eugenol base can be mixed thickly, rolled into a very small ball, and packed into the preparation using a very small amalgam plugger or an old explorer that has the tip cut off.

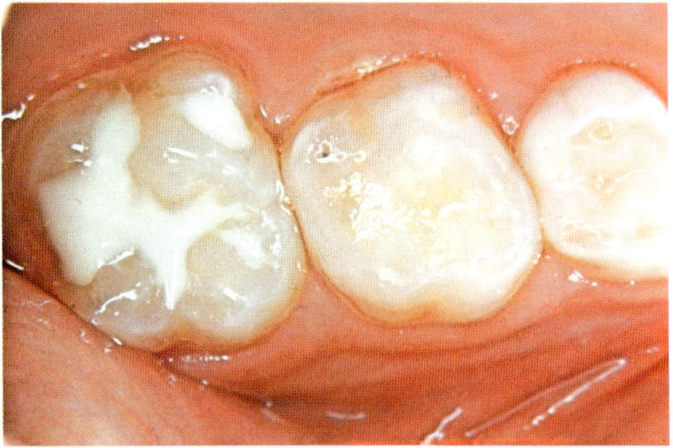

Fig. VIII-12   Patient C. M. Care must be taken, when applying dilute Concise to small preparations, that no air is trapped in the preparation. Applying an unfilled resin layer first, helps the flow of the material. Taking a very small amount of dilute Concise initially, and applying it to the wall of the preparation, usually allows the material to flow to the floor of the preparation.

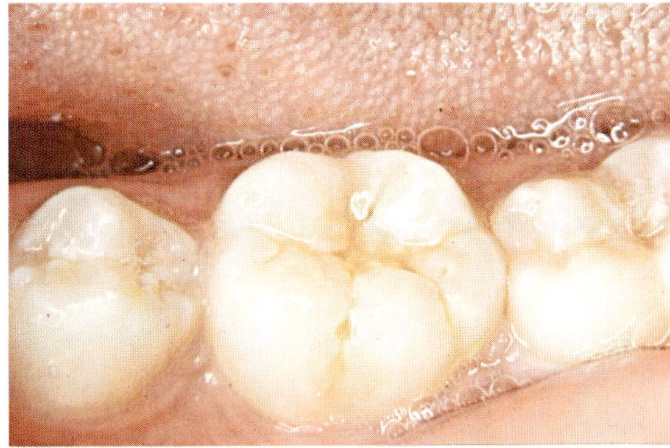

Fig. VIII-13   Patient L. P. The dilute Concise on this mandibular first permanent molar was applied 24 months previously. Preparations were made in the occlusal surface (2) and in the buccal groove (2). Wear was greatest at the top of the buccal groove but all preparations are covered and there is no leakage or secondary decay present.

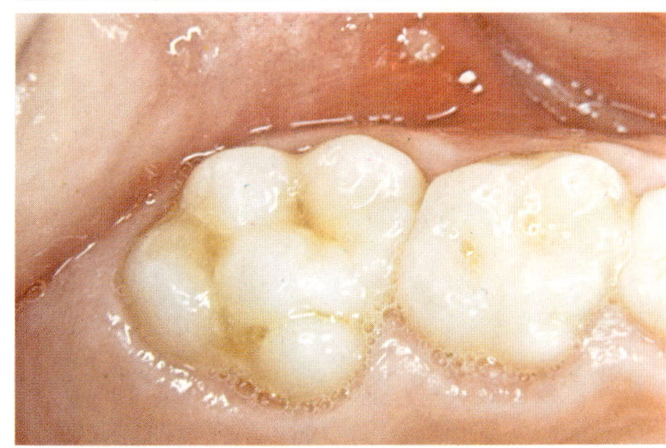

Fig. VIII-14   Patient D. F. This maxillary first permanent molar would have been severely weakened with an "extension for prevention" amalgam preparation. Twelve months previously dilute Concise was applied to all grooves. There was a single preparation made in the lingual groove for caries removal. No leakage or caries was detectable at recall.

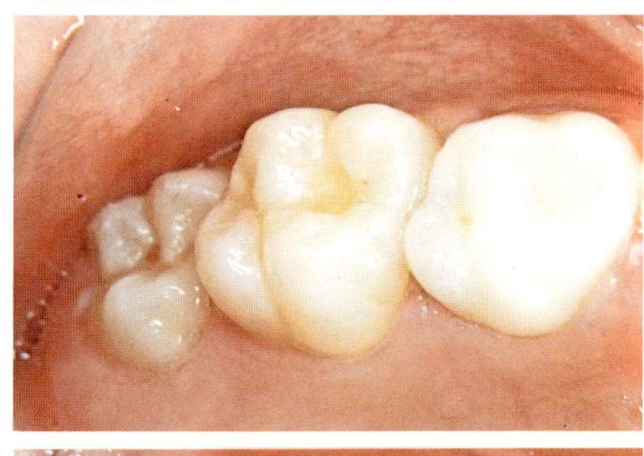

Fig. VIII-15   Patient J. M. The size of preparation on which dilute Concise can be used is limited. For larger preparations (Fig. VIII-19) filled resin should be used without dilution. Dilute Concise was applied to this preparation in the mesial portion of the occlusal groove. At 12 months the resin has worn down to a stage where addition of material is necessary.

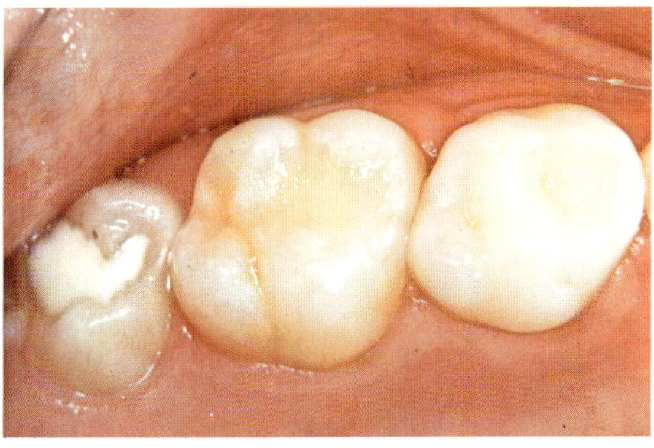

Fig. VIII-16   Patient J. M. The surface of the old dilute Concise was freshened up using a 7408 composite finishing bur (Fig. VII-5) and the enamel margins were re-etched. Concise was applied on top of Enamel Bond.

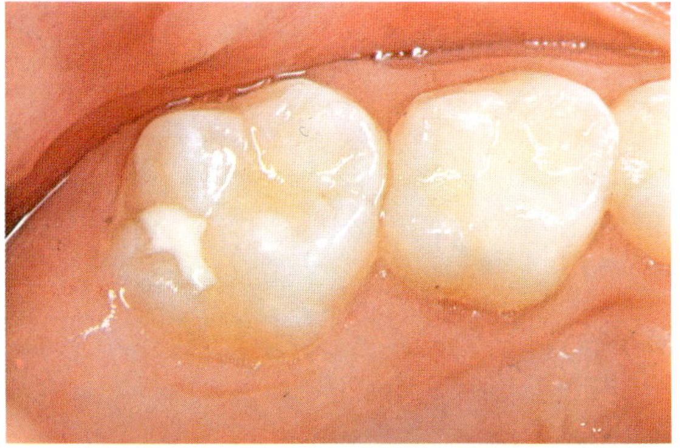

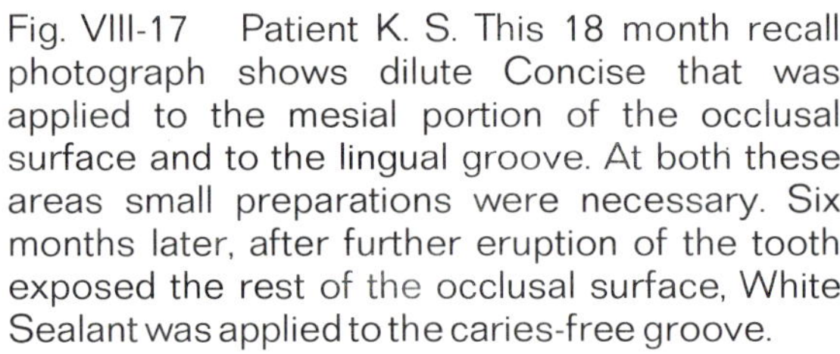

Fig. VIII-17   Patient K. S. This 18 month recall photograph shows dilute Concise that was applied to the mesial portion of the occlusal surface and to the lingual groove. At both these areas small preparations were necessary. Six months later, after further eruption of the tooth exposed the rest of the occlusal surface, White Sealant was applied to the caries-free groove.

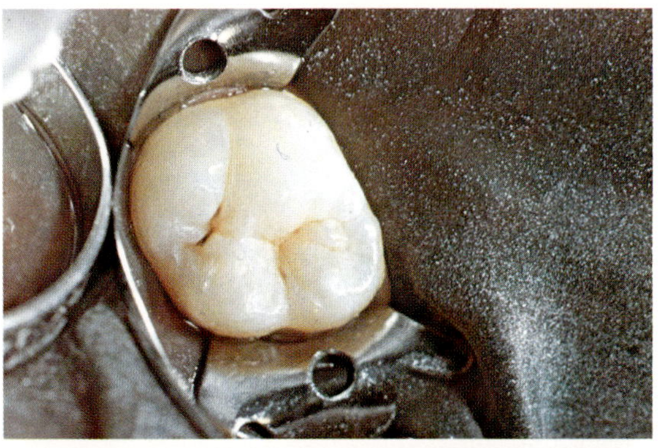

Fig. VIII-18   Patient M. M. With grooves such as this, it is sometimes hard to tell just how large the preparation will become. If x-ray indicates occlusal caries, rubber dam isolation should be utilized.

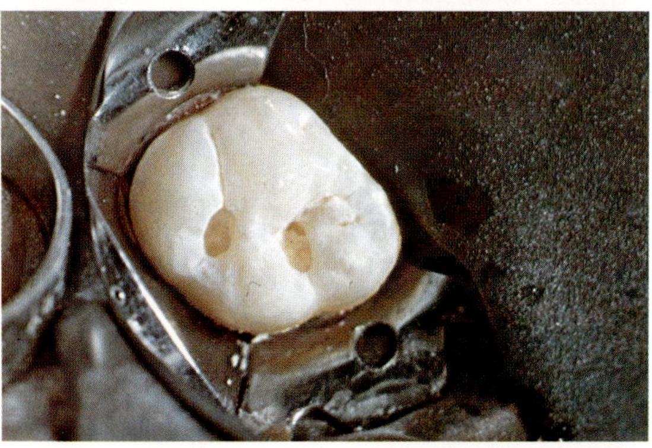

Fig. VIII-19   Patient M. M. Very careful examination of the preparation is necessary to assure that no caries has been left in the tooth laterally under the enamel surface. Calcium hydroxide base (Procal) has been applied and the surface etched. An amalgam preparation would have to be considerably more extensive to incorporate the rest of the occlusal grooves.

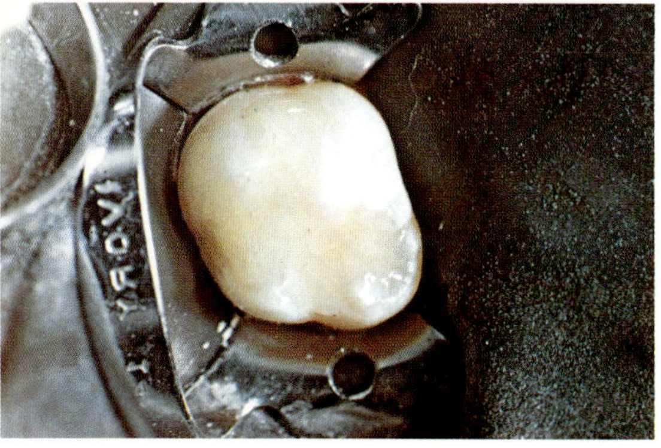

Fig. VIII-20   Patient M. M. After application of an unfilled resin layer (Enamel Bond) the radiopaque Concise is applied with a syringe. The syringe tip is placed at the base of the preparation. Thus filling takes place from the floor up, to avoid trapping air. All remaining pits and fissures are covered with composite. After removal of the rubber dam, occlusion must be checked with articulating paper.

References

1. *Asmussen, E.:*
Penetration of restorative resins into acid etched enamel. IADR abstract no. 349, February, 1977.

2. *Bodecker, C. F.:*
Enamel fissure eradication. NYSJD 30: April 64, 149–154.

3. *Buonocore, M. G.:*
The Use of Adhesives in Dentistry. Charles C. Thomas, Publisher, Springfield, Illinois, p. 257, 1975.

4. *Dogon, I. L.:*
Studies demonstrating the need for an intermediary resin of low viscosity for the acid etch technique. Proceedings of an International Symposium on the Acid Etch Technique. *Silverstone, L. M.* and *Dogon, I. L.* (Eds.), North Central Publishing Company, St. Paul, Minnesota, pp. 100–118, 1975.

5. *Dreyer Jorgensen, K.:*
The adaptation of composite and noncomposite resins to acid etched enamel surfaces. Proceedings of an International Symposium on the Acid Etch Technique. *Silverstone, L. M.* and *Dogon, I. L.* (Eds.), North Central Publishing Company, St. Paul, Minnesota, pp. 93–99, 1975.

6. *Forsten, L.:*
Effect of different factors on the marginal seal of composites. IADR abstract no. 427, February, 1977.

7. *Hinding, J. H.* and *Buonocore, M. G.:*
The effects of varying the application protocol on the retention of pit and fissure sealant: A 2-year clinical study. JADA 89: 127–131, 1974.

8. *Hyatt, T. P.:*
Prophylactic odontotomy: the cutting into the tooth for the prevention of disease. The Dental Cosmos, pp. 234–241, 1923.

9. *Mohammed, H., Schoen, F. J.* and *Burrell, E. R.:*
A simple comparative adhesion test method for composite resins. IADR abstract no. 350, February, 1977.

10. *Raadal, M.:*
Mikroretensjon av plastfyllingsmaterialer paa syreetset emalje. Den Norske Tannlaegeforenings Tidende. 10: 404–413, 1975.

11. *Raadal, M.:*
Personal Communication.

12. *Simonsen, R. J.:*
Acid Etch as a Preventive Technique in Dentistry. Chapter 18, in A Textbook of Preventive Dentistry. *Caldwell, R. C.* and *Stallard, R. E.* (Eds.). W. B. Saunders, Philadelphia, Pennsylvania, 1977.

13. *Simonsen, R. J.* and *Stallard, R. E.:*
Sealant-restorations utilizing a diluted filled resin: one year results. Quintessence Int. 6: 77–84, 1977.

14. *Silverstone, L. M.:*
Personal Communication.

15. *Ulvestad, H.:*
Clinical trials with fissure sealant materials in Scandinavia. Proceedings of an International Symposium on the Acid Etch Technique. *Silverstone, L. M.* and *Dogon, I. L.* (Eds.). North Central Publishing Company, St. Paul, Minnesota, pp. 165–175, 1975.

16. *Ulvestad, H.:*
A 24-month evaluation of fissure sealing with a diluted composite material. Scand. J. Dent. Res. 84: 51–55, 1976a.

17. *Ulvestad, H.:*
Evaluation of fissure sealing with a diluted composite sealant and an UV-light polymerized sealant after 36 months observation. Scand. J. Dent. Res. 84: 401–403, 1976b.

18. *Ulvestad, H.:*
Personal Communication.

Chapter 9

Splinting of Traumatic Injuries

Trauma to the anterior portion of the face frequently involves the incisor teeth. Coronal fractures (in varying degrees of severity), root fractures and mobility, are frequent sequelae to accidents involving the teeth. For traumatized teeth to have the best chance of healing, some support in the form of a splint is usually indicated.

Splinting of mobile teeth has been reported as early as the 8th century B. C., when the Etruscans used wire ligatures and gold bands to stabilize mobile teeth.[3] Wire ligatures are still in frequent use today for splinting. Other methods of splinting include using acrylic and orthodontic bands. All of these methods, however, involve a certain amount of post-traumatic manipulation of the teeth for fabrication of the splint. It is felt that elimination of tooth movement after injury may well be the most important criterion for successful splinting of traumatized teeth.

Buonocore's[4] initial paper dealing with the bonding of acrylic to acid-conditioned tooth enamel, has led to tremendous changes in the practice of dentistry, as have been documented in the preceeding chapters. The multiple uses of the acid etch system and the progress in the development of dental composite resins, has led to a method of splinting that is easier, faster to apply, less disturbing to the teeth and ultimately less costly to the accident victim than previous methods.

The goal in splinting traumatized teeth is to stabilize them for a period of time, to allow healing and to prevent further damage to the pulp and periodontal structures. Certain requirements for a successful splint were defined by *Andreasen*[1] in 1972.

1. It should allow direct application in the mouth without delay due to laboratory procedures.
2. It should not traumatize the tooth during application.
3. It should immobilize the injured tooth in a normal position.
4. It should provide adequate fixation throughout the entire period of immobilization.
5. It should neither damage the gingiva nor predispose to caries.
6. It should allow endodontic therapy if needed.
7. Preferably it should fulfill esthetic demands.

The types of traumatic splinting available at that time were:

1. Orthodontic band-acrylic splint
2. Interdental wiring
3. Arch bar
4. Acrylic splint
5. Cast silver crown splint

None of these splints fulfills all the requirements defined by *Andreasen*. Use of the acid etched splint does enable all of the requirements to be met.

Diagnosis

Diagnosing the necessity for splinting can be the most important step for the future health of traumatized teeth. Since an acid etch splint is easy to apply, and should cause very little disturbance of even a very busy office schedule, there is no reason for not applying a splint if any of the following indications are seen:

1. Root Fracture:

Radiographic diagnosis of root fracture can be somewhat difficult unless periodontal hemorrhaging, or the force of the blow, has separated the fragments. If a root fracture is suspected (from mobility), several radiographs should be taken at different angles to enhance the chances of detecting the fracture. Sometimes slight labial or lingual pressure on the tooth while the radiograph is being taken will disclose an otherwise invisible root fracture.

2. Subluxation (excessive mobility):

The dentist should be familiar with the normal mobility of erupting teeth in the various stages of eruption in order to be able to judge the extent of damage to traumatized teeth. Mobility is probably one of the surest indicators of potential traumatic sequelae, and no patient should be dismissed from an office without some supportive treatment if the teeth have become mobile after trauma. Extrusive luxation (partial evulsion) can be diagnosed by increased width of the periodontal ligament on x-ray.

3. Periodontal Hemorrhage:

Any sign of bleeding from the periodontal structures (not to be confused with extra-oral and intra-oral soft tissue wounds), is an indication that the tooth has received a severe blow. Necessity for splinting is determined by the amount of hemorrhage, eruptive stage of the tooth and mobility.

4. Displacement or Evulsion:

Permanent teeth can be successfully repositioned and splinted even after severe displacement or evulsion. Post healing endodontic therapy is almost inevitable in such cases. Evulsion and replantation criteria are not described here, although one method of splinting shown (Case No. 4) does involve an evulsed tooth.

Technique

Step 1.

Initially the teeth should be cleaned with pumice unless severely mobile teeth are involved. (It is more important to minimize the post-traumatic manipulation than it is to ensure clean enamel surfaces for etching.)

Step 2.

The enamel areas to be bonded should be dried and orthophosphoric acid applied for 60 seconds. The strength of the acid used will vary with the product used. The 3M Concise Enamel Bond utilizes 37% orthophosphoric acid and also contains small sponges for acid application. The acid falls within the ideal range (30%–40%) quoted by *Silverstone*.[11] Isolation during etching is important and should be as effective as possible. It must be remembered that primary consideration should still be given to minimal post-traumatic manipulation. Therefore, rubber dam is contraindicated for traumatic splint isolation, as displacement of mobile teeth may result from the tension in the rubber dam.

Step 3.

Thorough washing and drying after etching is essential. The acid and its precipitates must be washed off, using water (units that mix mouthwash in their water spray should not be used). The etched area must then be maintained as dry as possible until the resin can be applied. This may be difficult in some cases, due to hemorrhage from soft tissue or periodontal ligament injury (Figs. IX-6 and 9).

Step 4.

Immediately after drying, the unfilled resin layer should be applied. A fresh sponge, held in a lockable cotton plier, is excellent for applying a thin layer of unfilled resin. The necessity for using an intermediate layer has been both supported and attacked in the literature. *Dreyer Jorgensen,*[7] *Raadal,*[10] *Asmussen*[2] and *Ulvestad*[12] all expressed belief that as much resin penetration (producing resin "tags" for retention) into etched enamel is obtained using the filled resin, as with the unfilled resin.

Dogon[6] found, and *Forsten*[8] confirmed, that the intermediate resin layer decreased microleakage. Increased bond strength, using an intermediate resin layer, has been found by *Buonocore*[5] and *Mohammed, Schoen and Burrell*[9].

Step 5.

The filled resin (3M Concise) is added into the embrasures with a syringe (Centrix C-R) immediately after applying the unfilled resin. Wooden wedges can be used to prevent the resin from flowing onto the gingival papillae, but great care must be taken not to displace mobile teeth with the pressure of a wedge. It is usually best to let the resin flow where it may and trim it away from the gingiva after polymerization. When using Concise for splints, it is best to mix more of the catalyst paste (yellow jar—paste B) than universal, (orange jar—paste A), rather than equal amounts. This will increase the polymerization and working times. Where esthetics are of importance, the material can be applied more to the lingual than the labial.

Step 6.

Any excess material can be trimmed away, using high-speed fluted finishing burs, (7901 FG or 7408 FG, Midwest American).

Case History No. 1

A 10 year-old boy reported to the Dental Clinic the day after sustaining a severe blow to the upper central incisors during a hockey game. A periapical radiograph indicated root fractures in the middle one-third of the roots of both central incisors. Both teeth were very mobile and the radiograph showed the root fragments had separated, from periodontal ligament hemorrhage into the fractured area.

A splint was applied, using the 3M Concise Enamel Bond System. Any of the commercially available resins can be used in a similar manner. Labial and lingual views of this procedure are shown in Figures IX-1 and 2.

Three weeks later, these teeth received another blow, again during a hockey game. The filled composite resin fractured between the central incisors. The weak link in such splints is not the bonded area between the enamel surface and composite resin, but the inherent strength of the filled composite resin. Thus, for longer spans between splinted teeth, further support is needed, as will be seen in Case No. 3. Had the patient's teeth not been splinted at the time of receiving the second blow, the damage could have been far more severe, as the splint undoubtedly absorbed much of the impact.

The splint was removed after 24 weeks, (Fig. IX-3), and the patient was checked again three months after splint removal.

In this case, the splint was utilized for six months, due to the severity of the initial injury and the fact that further trauma was sustained. Generally, splinting for more than 3–6 weeks is not necessary. In severe cases, where longer term splinting is desired, part of the splint (i.e., lateral to central bonds) can be removed, while leaving the most important bond (for example between the central incisors) in place. This patient was seen 18 months post-trauma (Fig. IX-4). There was no sign of any developing pathosis. All anterior teeth tested positive with an electric pulp tester.

Case History No. 2

An 11 year-old boy was seen on an emergency basis after a weekend skiing accident. Dental care was commenced after suturing the soft tissue damage (Fig. IX-5). In this case, the metal edge of a heavy downhill ski caught the boy across the mouth, resulting in evulsion of the upper right lateral, fracture of upper right central, fracture of lower right incisors, evulsion of lower left central and fracture and severe displacement of the lower left lateral (Fig. IX-6). All fractured teeth had pulpal exposures large enough to necessitate endodontic therapy. Neither of the evulsed teeth were found at the accident site.

The challenge here was to stabilize the displaced lower left lateral incisor and retain it as a bridge abutment for future prosthetic restoration. After removal of vital pulp tissue and placement of a small pledget of cotton with medication in the pulp chamber (this was only to avoid any pain from pulpal necrosis while the splint was in place), the tooth was repositioned with finger pressure and splinted to the cuspid. Etching was extremely difficult, as the soft tissue hemorrhaged and saliva was continually contaminating the etched surfaces.

Enamel Bond and Concise were applied with the thought that, should the splint fail, it could be replaced after soft tissue healing, when conditions for etching would be markedly

improved. Fortunately, this was not necessary, and after recall at three weeks (Fig. IX-7) the patient was referred for endodontic therapy which was completed without removing the splint. The splint was removed for prosthetic completion of the case eight weeks after application, at which time the lateral incisor was firmly in place. Figure IX-8 shows the same case 18 months after completion. The displaced lateral has been successfully used as a bridge abutment, with no radiographic evidence of any pathosis.

Case History No. 3

A seven year-old boy with partially erupted upper central incisors sustained a blow to both upper central incisors, resulting in fractures of both mesio-incisal corners. Hemorrhage was present, both from a gingival laceration above the right central incisor, and from the periodontal ligament around the same tooth. Although both centrals were damaged, the left central had normal mobility for its eruptive stage, whereas the right central had severely excessive mobility and splinting was definitely indicated. Periapical radiography showed no apparent root or alveolar bone fracture. Both teeth had wide-open apices, indicating that the prognosis for healing after stabilization would be good.

Two problems were immediately apparent. The hemorrhage, from the periodontal ligament space and the soft tissue injury, would be difficult to control and would interfere with etching. Secondly, the wide space between the centrals and the absence of the lateral incisors (one was exfoliating; the other had to be extracted) make splinting, such as in Case No. 1, impossible. The problem was simply resolved by cutting a small length of arch wire (.81 mm, .032″) and slightly bending it to conform to the anterior arch curvature.

One joint at a time was bonded (Fig. IX-9). The enamel surface of each central was etched, as previously described, and the resin added liberally around the wire. The hemorrhage from the periodontal ligament injury did not contaminate the etched enamel until all the composite had been applied. However, there was contamination of the composite along the upper edge immediately after application and prior to the composite polymerizing (Fig. IX-10). This did not have any effect on retention.

The splint was removed after periapical radiography at 6-week recall showed no developing problems (Fig. IX-11). Stability was normal and mesial corners were restored at the same appointment, using the technique described in Chapter 3 (Fig. IX-12).

Case History No. 4

For splinting across a larger span than a diastema, the stainless steel space bar, (as designed for space maintenance and described in Chapter 10), is used.

A seven year-old girl was brought to the emergency clinic after a bicycle accident. The upper left central incisor was brought along in a plastic bag, as it had been evulsed and then recovered at the accident site.

Replanting of the tooth was attempted, despite the time lag since trauma was over one hour (replanting stands the greatest chance of success if it can be accomplished within 30 minutes).

The two central incisors are first bonded together, using the same technique as for Case History No. 1. A stainless steel space bar is adapted to the labial surface of the central incisor and the deciduous cuspid, using a three-jaw wire bending plier. The two holes at each end of the space bar allow for penetration of composite and attachment of the bar. The bonding surfaces are then etched, (one at a time), and unfilled resin and filled resin applied around the end of the bar. Completing one bond at a time allows the operator to hold the bar firmly in place on the other tooth, during polymerization of the first bond. This assures that the bar is placed in the correct position, and is not moved during polymerization.

These four cases illustrate some of the most common ways that the acid etch technique can be used for traumatic splinting. There are obviously innumerable variations on the technique. The main benefit of the technique is that the splint can be applied rapidly, with no post-trauma movement of the damaged teeth, thus increasing the chances of successful healing.

Semi-permanent or permanent splints for periodontal support can be similarly made, the design depending on the length of the span and degree of support needed. Seldom, if ever, is tooth preparation necessary or justifiable for retention.

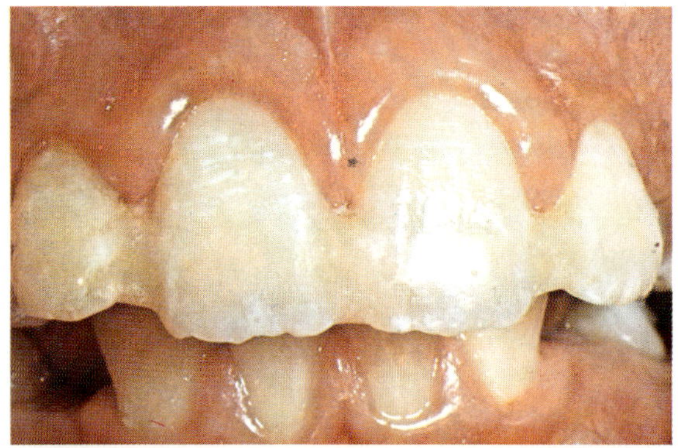

Fig. IX-1   Patient T. Y. This patient severely fractured both central incisor roots in the apical one-third of the roots during a hockey game. The interproximal areas of the four anterior teeth were etched and Enamel Bond followed by Concise was applied. In this fashion the teeth can be rapidly splinted, with little or no further movement and irritation to the damaged teeth.

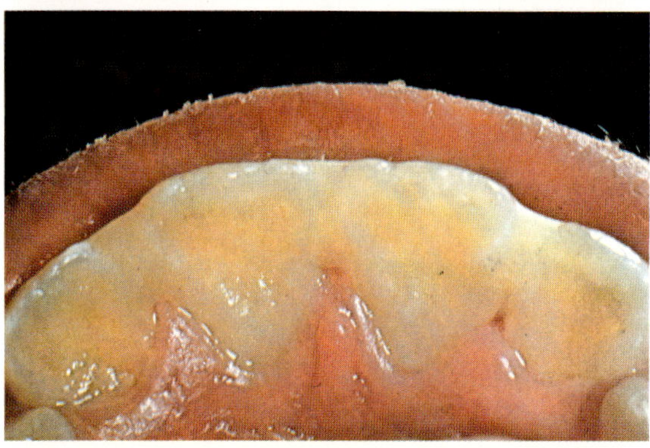

Fig. IX-2   Patient T. Y. The lingual view of the splint seen in Figure IX-1. The lingual surfaces can be used more than the labial for stabilization, if esthetics are important and the occlusion permits it.

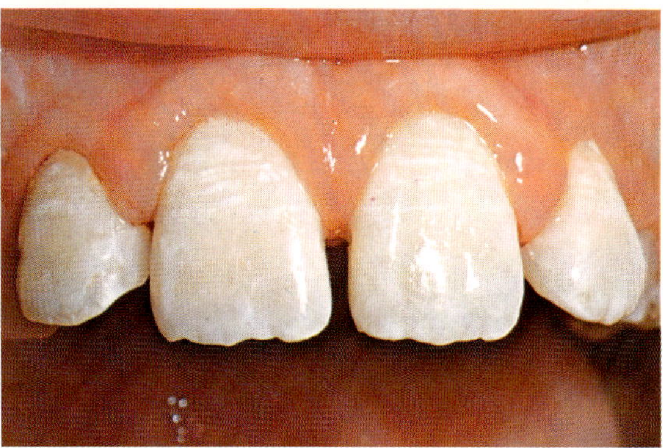

Fig. IX-3   Patient T. Y. After splint removal the teeth responded positively to an electric pulp test. The splint in this case was in place much longer than normally necessary, (about 6 months), due to the severity of the injury and to the fact that a second blow was received later in the hockey season breaking the splint (within the composite) between the central incisors.

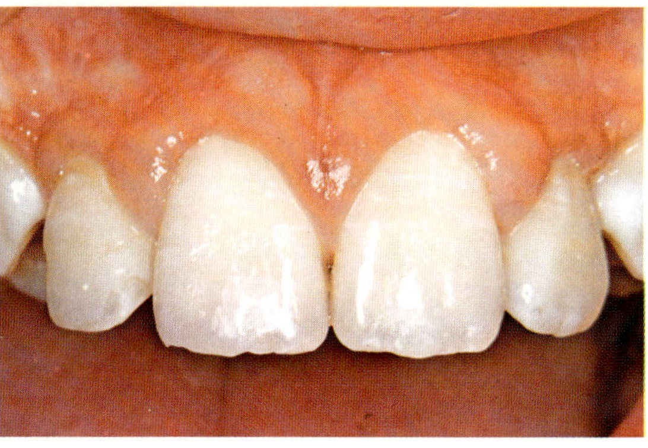

Fig. IX-4   Patient T. Y. One year after splint removal the teeth are still testing vital and are asymptomatic.

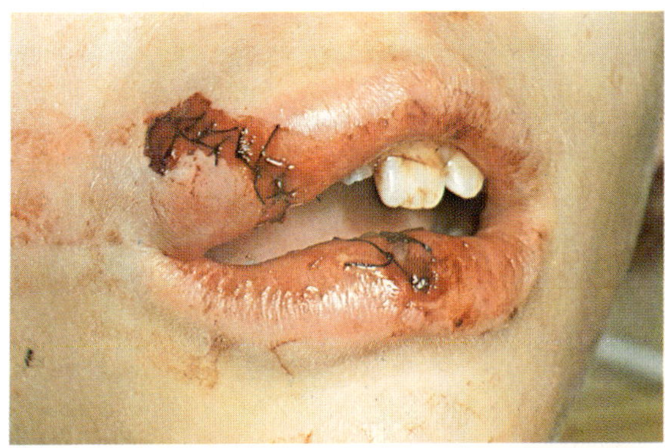

Fig. IX-5   Patient J. Ba. A skiing accident resulted in this lip laceration and the evulsion and fracture of several anterior teeth. The heavy metal edge of a downhill ski caught this 11 year-old boy across the mouth.

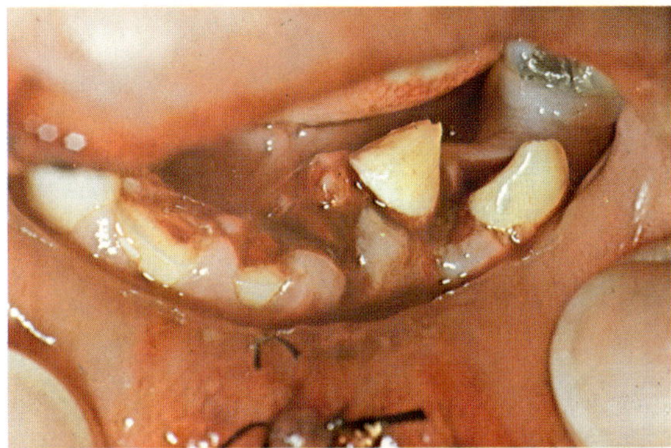

Fig. IX-6   Patient J. Ba. After suturing the soft tissue, attention was turned to the teeth. One tooth, the mandibular left lateral incisor was severely lingually displaced in addition to being fractured. The adjacent central was evulsed and both other incisors fractured with pulpal exposures. Emergency endodontics was performed but the main challenge was to save the lingually displaced lateral incisor.

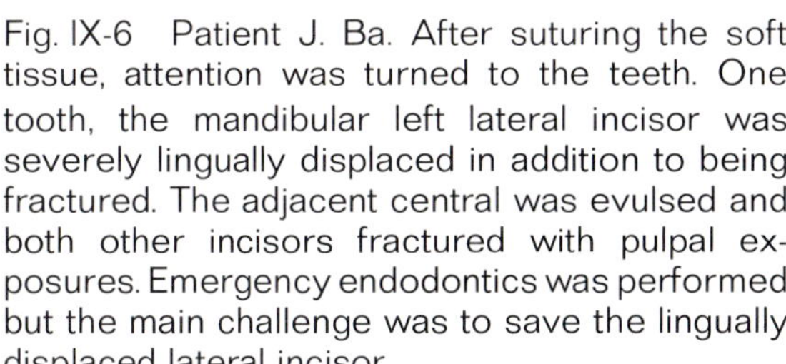

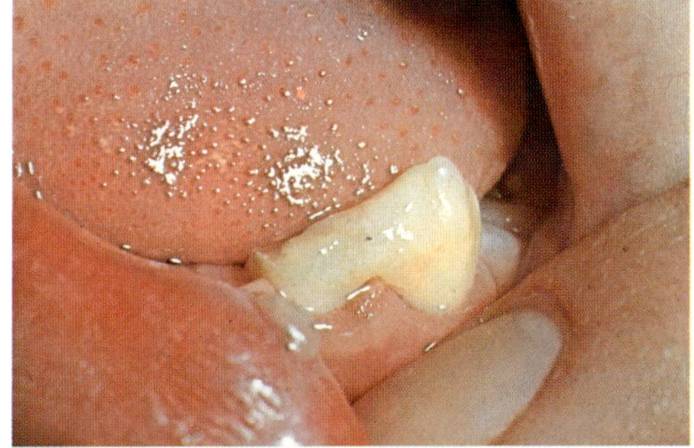

Fig. IX-7   Patient J. Ba. Despite less than optimal conditions for bonding, the tooth was repositioned and splinted to the cuspid using Concise. This 3-week recall photograph shows the splint firmly in place. Endodontic therapy was completed without removing the splint which was left in place for a further five weeks. The lateral was successfully used as an abutment for a fixed bridge, replacing the missing central incisor.

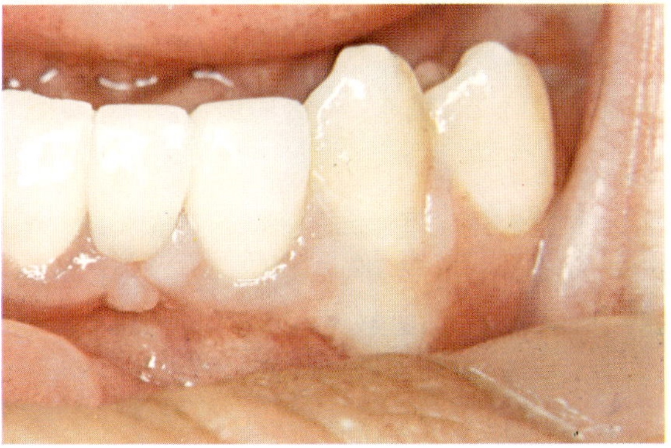

Fig. IX-8   Patient J. Ba. 18 months after the original injury the lateral is still functioning perfectly. No other method of splinting could have successfully repositioned and held firmly in place the lateral incisor with so little post-trauma irritation. Rapid application of acid etch splints can save many teeth previously thought impossible to maintain in the mouth.

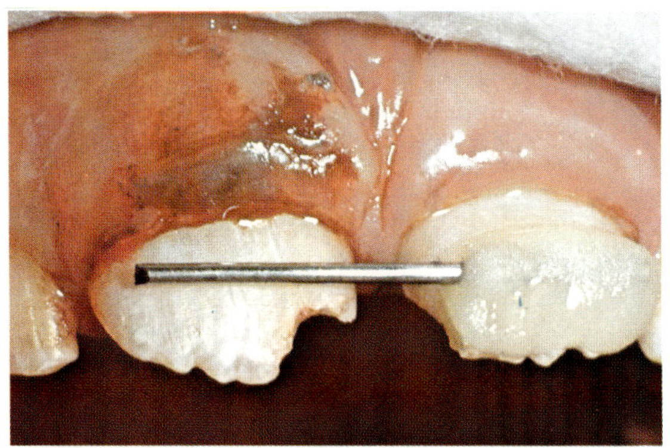

Fig. IX-9   Patient J. Bi. When the trauma occurs as the teeth are erupting, as in the case of this subluxed maxillary right central incisor, it is frequently impossible to use the type of splint used in Figure IX-1. A 0.81 mm wire was slightly bent to conform to the curvature of the arch and bonded to the uninjured central incisor with Concise.

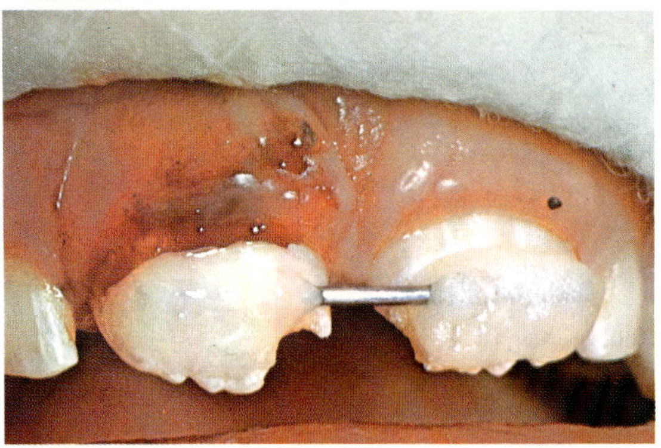

Fig. IX-10   Patient J. Bi. Hemorrhage from the soft tissue injury was kept away from the bonding site as much as possible, but it did contaminate the composite before polymerization. This did not affect the successful retention of the splint. Prognosis for healing of newly erupted teeth after trauma is good, as the wide open apices ensure a plentiful blood supply.

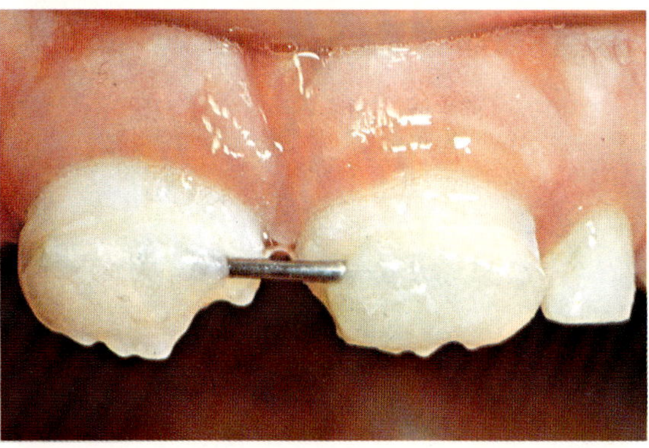

Fig. IX-11   Patient J. Bi. Six weeks after trauma the splint was removed using diamonds for gross removal of composite, and the 7901 FG carbide finishing bur (Midwest American) for delicate removal of the remaining composite. The mesio-incisal corners of the central incisors were then restored with Concise.

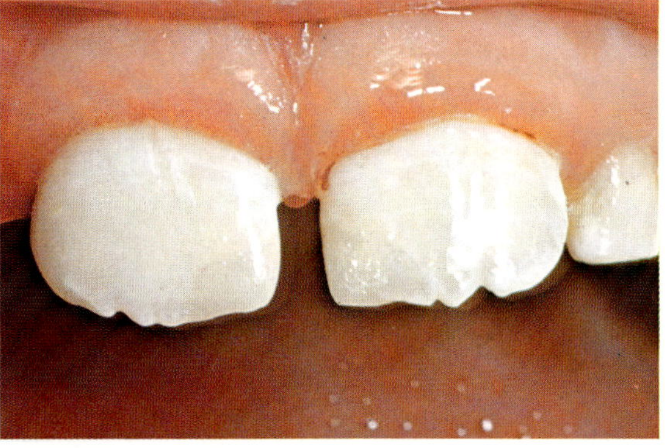

Fig. IX-12   Patient J. B. The completed case after splint removal and restoration of incisal fractures. At this time the right and left central incisors had similar degrees of mobility, consistent with their eruptive stage.

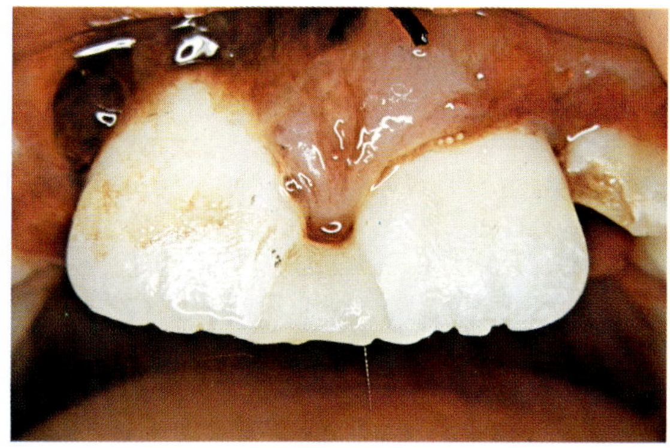

Fig. IX-13   Patient C. P. Acid etch splinting is also useful where replantation is attempted. The maxillary left central incisor has just been replanted and bonded to the right central. This should be done as rapidly as possible to get initial stabilization. Further stabilization is, however, needed, and the lateral is only partially erupted (and fractured) eliminating its use.

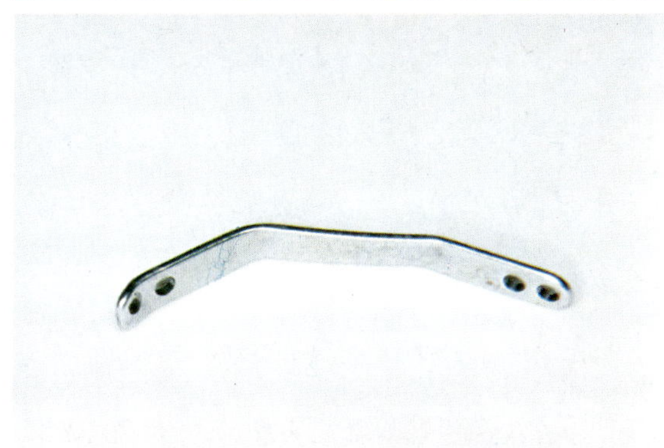

Fig. IX-14   Patient C. P. In order to span the gap to the stable deciduous cuspid, a space bar, (Chapter X), was adapted to the labial surfaces of cuspid and central. Holes in the ends of the stainless steel band allow the composite to mechanically lock around the band.

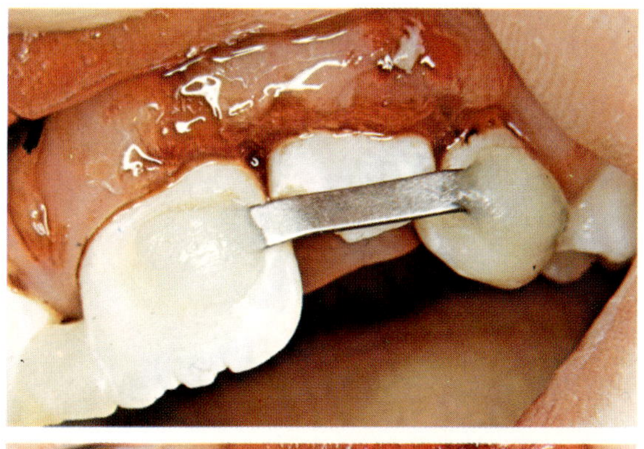

Fig. IX-15   Patient C. P. The bonding to permanent central and deciduous cuspid is now complete and the central incisor is stable.

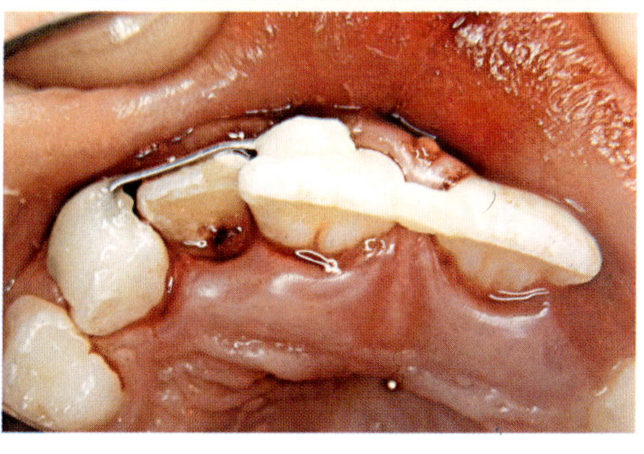

Fig. IX-16   Patient C. P. Incisal view of the central to cuspid splint utilizing the stainless steel space bar. The splint should be left in place for 3–6 weeks (*Andreasen*[1], p. 212). The replanted tooth should be closely followed with regular periapical radiographs to watch for possible, (probable), root resorption.

References

1. *Andreasen, J. O.:*
Traumatic Injuries of the Teeth. Munksgaard, Copenhagen, Denmark, 1972.

2. *Asmussen, E.:*
Penetration of restorative resins into acid etched enamel. IADR abstract no. 349, February, 1977.

3. *Baumhammers, A.:*
Temporary and Semi-permanent Splinting. Charles C. Thomas, Publisher, Springfield, Illinois, 1971.

4. *Buonocore, M. G.:*
A simple method of increasing the adhesion of acrylic filling materials to enamel surfaces. J. Dent. Res. 34: 849–853, 1955.

5. *Buonocore, M. G.:*
The Use of Adhesives in Dentistry, p. 247. Charles C. Thomas, Publisher, Springfield, Illinois, 1975.

6. *Dogon, I. L.:*
Studies demonstrating the need for an intermediary resin of low viscosity for the acid etch technique. Proceedings of an International Symposium on the Acid Etch Technique. *Silverstone, L. M.* and *Dogon, I. L.* (Eds.) . North Central Publishing Co., St. Paul, Minnesota, pp. 100–118, 1975.

7. *Dreyer Jorgensen, K.:*
The adaptation of composite and non-composite resins to acid etched enamel surfaces. Proceedings of an International Symposium on the Acid Etch Technique. *Silverstone, L. M.* and *Dogon, I. L.* (Eds.). North Central Publishing Co., St. Paul, Minnesota, pp. 93–99, 1975.

8. *Forsten, L.:*
Effect of different factors on the marginal seal of composites. IADR abstract no. 427, February, 1977.

9. *Mohammed, H., Schoen, F. J.* and *Burrell, E. R.:*
A simple comparative adhesion test method for composite resins. IADR abstract no. 350, February, 1977.

10. *Raadal, M.:*
Mikroretensjon av plastfyllingsmaterialer paa syreetset emalje. Den Norske Tannlaegeforenings Tidende. 10: 404–413, 1975.

11. *Silverstone, L. M.*
Fissure sealants: Laboratory Studies. Caries Res. 8: 2–26, 1974.

12. *Ulvestad, H.:*
Personal Communication.

Chapter 10

Space Maintenance

Space maintenance has traditionally been a multiple-visit procedure requiring banding, impressioning and several steps in the laboratory manufacture of the typical band-and-loop appliance (Figs. X-1 and 4) prior to seating and cementing. Various problems that can arise with these appliances are seen in Figures X-1 to 5. With the use of the acid etch principle and either ultraviolet or chemically curing composite systems, simple space maintainers can be more readily made, applied with less cost to the patient, and retained with overall better gingival health to the tissue around the abutment teeth.

If the principles of bonding composite to enamel are followed carefully, the bond will last the months or years necessary for holding the space prior to eruption of the permanent succedaneous tooth. The bonded unit will be very stable and will eliminate the problem of the loop slipping below the contact point of the abutment tooth (Fig. X-3) or of chronic loss of the appliance (Fig. X-2).

This chapter will not concern itself with the diagnosis of space maintenance necessity. It will merely describe a simplified clinical technique for holding space.

Technique

In initial attempts at using the acid etch system for space maintenance, 0.81 mm (.032") wire was bent with loops at each end and bonded to abutment teeth. A similar technique was used by *Swaine* and *Wright*[2] who found a 70% success rate (based on retention at 6 months) for their cases completed in this manner.

In an attempt to improve the quality of, and ease of adapting the bonding metal, this author approached the 3M Company, St. Paul, Minnesota, with the idea for a metal bar space maintainer. The 3M Company made some samples and the one chosen had two perforations at each end of a 20 mm long strip of stainless steel, 0.48 mm thick and 2 2 mm wide (Fig. X-7). This stainless steel strip is preferable to a .032" wire for several reasons:

1. The strip is easier to adapt, particularly to short clinical crowns.
2. The strip, having a width of 2 mm, cannot be inadvertantly bent by a sharp chewing force.
3. The strip is thinner (0.48 mm) than .032" wire (0.81 mm), thus allowing less bulky bonds.

Adaptation of the strip

A three-jaw wire bending plier is excellent for making the necessary bends at the ends of the strip in order for the strip to conform to the buccal or lingual anatomy of the abutment teeth. To avoid occlusal interferences, it is frequently desirable to bond maxillary strips to the buccal surfaces, and mandibular strips to the lingual surfaces, even though this makes access more difficult in the mandibular quadrants. The space maintainer will work equally well buccally or lingually. If esthetics are of importance, a lingually placed space maintainer is best.

As can be seen from Figure X-8, the strip can be made to closely conform to the anatomy of the tooth, thus assuring a uniform thickness of composite material between the strip and the tooth. *Buonocore*[1] stresses the importance of this "uniform adhesive thickness between bracket and tooth structure" when discussing the bonding of orthodontic brackets to teeth. This uniformity of bonded joints is far easier to achieve using the 3M stainless strips than .032" wire. If the clinical crown is very short, the strip can be cut down without loss of strength or retention, to avoid the unnecessary irritation of gingival tissue from composite resin material.

Bonding

Swaine and *Wright*[2] made use of the rubber dam for isolation when bonding .032" wire space maintainers. Undoubtedly the advantages of rubber dam use far outweigh its disadvantages. However, in a study, the results of which will be presented in this chapter, it was hoped to show that successful bonds could, with care, be made without rubber dam isolation. Most practitioners still do not use the rubber dam regularly and it is, therefore, pertinent to present a technique and its results that will give practitioners a realistic impression of the results they may expect. Cotton rolls and Hygoformic saliva ejector (particularly for mandibular lingual bonding) were, therefore, frequently used for isolation. Few problems with salivary contamination were encountered using this method of isolation. Use of the rubber dam, however, invariably makes isolation much easier (Fig. X-10).

Enamel surfaces to be etched were pumiced to remove plaque and enamel pellicle. A rubber prophylaxis cup is adequate for smooth surface cleaning, although a brush may be needed on surfaces containing a groove, such as the buccal surface of the mandibular first permanent molars.

In the first attempts at bonding space maintainers, both joints were completed at one time. After etching permanent enamel for 60 seconds, and deciduous enamel for 120 seconds (with 37% orthophosphoric acid), and thorough washing and drying, 3M Concise Brand Enamel Bond was applied to the etched surface. Concurrently, the filled composite Concise was mixed and then applied around the ends of the wire and also on top of the Enamel Bond layer. The wire was then held in place, using a lockable cotton pliers, until material had set. It was found, later, with the introduction of the stainless steel strip, that the strip could be more accurately placed, and more firmly held in place during bonding, if one bond was done at a time. Thus, the technique has been utilized of bonding the most accessible tooth first. Only the tooth surface to be bonded is etched initially, (to prevent contamination of the second tooth surface during bonding of the first tooth), great care being taken, as usual in any acid etch procedure, to avoid any salivary contamination of the etched surface prior to placement of the unfilled resin layer. Enamel Bond, followed by Concise, is then applied to the etched surface and one end of the stainless steel bar. The other end of the bar is firmly held in place while the composite polymerizes. In this way, the bar is certain to be bonded in the correct place and movement during polymerization is eliminated.

After completion of one bond, the other tooth can be etched and completed in a similar fashion (Figs. X-9 and 10). No failures have been found in the bonds completed in this manner. The one failure seen so far occurred in the first space maintainer placed, using the 3M strip, where both bonds were done together. This may have been a contributing factor to the loss, although it is thought that heavy occlusion was the main cause of failure.

Applying the acid and resin layer to the second tooth surface must be done carefully to assure penetration of both acid and resin to all enamel surfaces under the metal strip. The perforated ends of the strip make this easier, as well as aiding in retention. In all cases, the Centrix C-R syringe was used to apply the filled resin into the perforations and around the metal strip. Care should be taken to avoid approaching the gingiva with composite resin, if possible.

Finishing

Any excessive bulk of composite can be easily trimmed, using a highspeed fluted composite finishing bur. Particular attention was made to the composite towards the gingiva in order to eliminate any gingival irritation from composite flash. A glaze layer of 5% sub-micron filled resin was applied, after washing and drying, to provide a smoother surface for tongue or cheek tissues.

Lingual and trans-palatal arches

Adapting lingual arch wires into grooves on first permanent molars, and then etching and bonding them in place, also eliminates the use of orthodontic bands and laboratory fees in these space maintainers. A study model is taken and .032" (0.81 mm) wire adapted as needed. For maxillary trans-palatal arches, the ends of the wire are adapted into the occluso-lingual groove, which provides support against occlusal stresses for the space maintainer (Fig. X-15). For mandibular lingual arches, it is convenient to adapt the wire into the lingual groove and carry it 2–3 mm down the groove towards the central

fossa (Fig. X-14). This will aid in retention, as the wire will be supported against occlusal forces by the occlusal bend. The wire should be adapted along the middle ⅓ of the lingual surface, making certain to keep it away from the gingival margin to avoid irritation from the composite bond.

After adaptation on the cast, the arch can be bonded in no more time than it would take to cement the orthodontic bands. As in the case with the stainless steel strip space maintainer, it was found by trial and error to be easier to bond one tooth at a time. In the maxilla, this is simply accomplished by holding the wire in place on one tooth while bonding the other tooth (same technique as described previously). Alternatively, some water-based impression material can be placed around the wire in the palate. This will then hold the wire in place during bonding, and the impression material can be easily removed when bonding of both molars is complete.

In the mandibular arch, Hygoformic saliva ejectors are excellent for restraining the tongue, as well as removing saliva. It has been found beneficial to mix a little impression material or compound impression material first and use this to temporarily anchor the lingual arch wire to the lower anterior teeth in the desired position (Fig. X-16). This ensures that the wire is in the correct position for bonding and the impression material or compound can be easily cut away and flicked off the teeth after both permanent molars are bonded.

Such joints, as described here, are remarkably strong. This can be demonstrated during removal when the wire can be torqued considerably without having any effect on the bond itself. Removal of the bond is simply accomplished by grinding the composite to the wire, pulling off the wire, and then with a high-speed fluted composite finishing bur, gradually removing all of the composite down to the enamel surface. Using the high-speed dry, it is very clearly seen when the last

Clinical study

Type of Maintainer	Maxillary		Mandibular		Time in
	Placed	Lost	Placed	Lost	Place
3M Stainless Steel Strip	18	1*	17	0	12 months
Lingual arch			9	1**	12 months
Trans-palatal arch	6	0			12 months
3M Stainless Steel Strip	6	0	4	0	24 months
Lingual arch			4	0	24 months
Trans-palatal arch	3	0			24 months

* Lost 3 weeks after application   ** Lost 2 weeks after application

Note: The failures at 12 months are not included at 24 months. Unless composite wear causes loss of the appliance, any space maintainer that remains bonded for 3 months, probably will remain in place until it is removed.

layer of the composite is removed and tooth enamel is reached.

Examples of one-year (Fig. X-12) and two-year (Fig. X-20) space maintainers show the excellent performance of the acid etch bond.

The one failure with the stainless steel strip, seen at 12 months, was placed from the lingual of an upper deciduous cuspid to the lingual of an upper deciduous second molar. The maxillary lingual is not an ideal location, as considerable grinding to eliminate occlusal interferences, (mainly from the lower cuspid), is frequently necessary. It is believed inadequate occlusal relief was the main cause of the failure. The bond itself did not fail, as there was composite material left on both teeth at the bonding site. The fracture occurred within the filled composite material and it is noteworthy that the strength of such bonds is limited not by the strength of the bond itself, but by the inherent strength of the composite material used.

The one lingual arch failure before 12 months was placed on a child with a very large active tongue, profuse salivary flow and strong gag reflex. These types of problems lead to poor moisture control, and it was not therefore surprising, that conditions for successful bonding were not met.

The use of composite to bond space maintainers to enamel surfaces, has shown itself to be another beneficial adjunct of the acid etch technique. Many problems frequently encountered with conventional band-and-loop or lingual arches placed with orthodontic bands (particularly problems of cement washing out and the bands loosening) can be avoided by bonding.

As has been stressed in the previous chapters, the success of this technique is dependent totally on the quality of the clinical application. If the basic rules of clinical acid etch bonded composite are followed, this, and the other uses of the technique, will be of great satisfaction to both the practitioner and his patients.

The author is indebted to Dr. *Richard Joos* and Mr. *Jack Hood* of the 3M Company for their assistance in the development of the stainless steel space maintainer described here.

References

1. *Buonocore, M. G.:*
   The Use of Adhesives in Dentistry. Charles C. Thomas, Publisher, Springfield, Illinois, p. 25, 1975.

2. *Swaine, T. J.* and *Wright, G. Z.:*
   Direct bonding applied to space maintenance. J. Dent. Child. 6: 401–405, 1976.

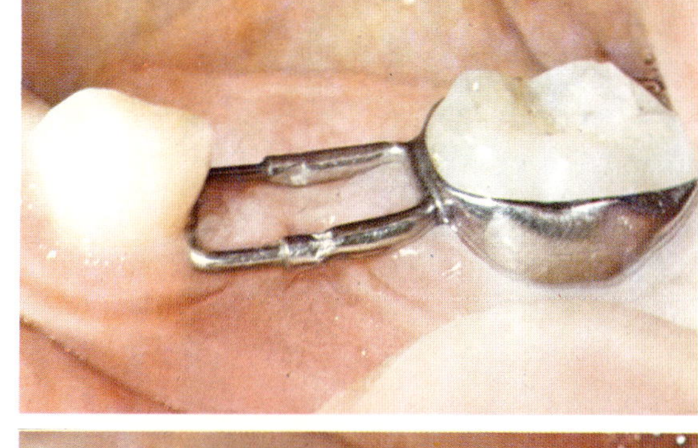

Fig. X-1   Patient J. R. The torque placed on space maintainers of this type during mastication, causes frequent loosening of the band and gingival irritation.

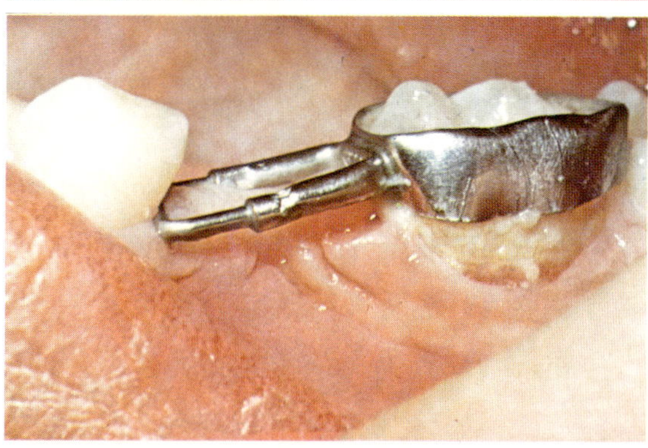

Fig. X-2   Patient J. R. While examining this patient, it was discovered that the space maintainer was loose. Underneath, a large amount of plaque and debris was found. The patient subsequently reported having had the band re-cemented on four different occasions prior to the family moving to Minnesota. The space maintainer was removed and replaced in 15 minutes according to the technique described here.

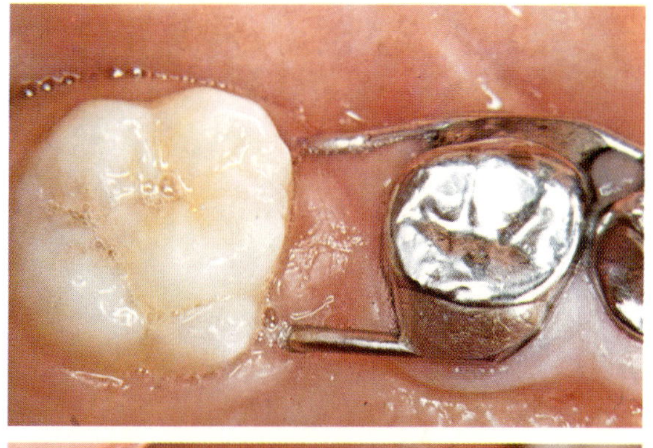

Fig. X-3   Patient A. W. Tipping of teeth over space maintainer loops causes the loop to end up sub-gingivally, sometimes, (as in this case), half-way down the root. This not only is a chronic irritant to the periodontal structures, but it also negates the purpose of the space maintainer.

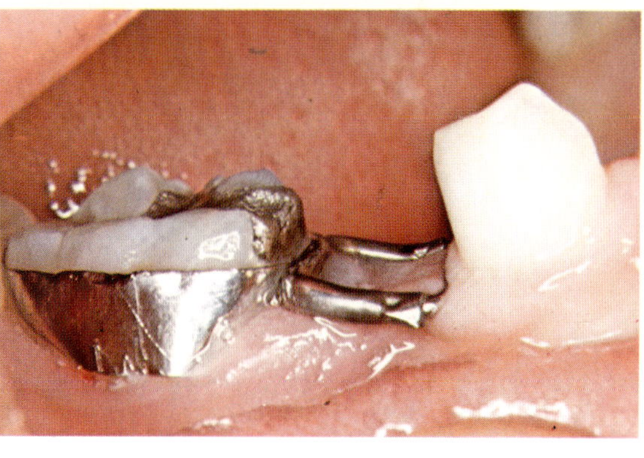

Fig. X-4   Patient J. S. The forces of mastication have pushed the loop into the gingival tissues causing chronic irritation. The band around the first permanent molar is also a site of gingival irritation.

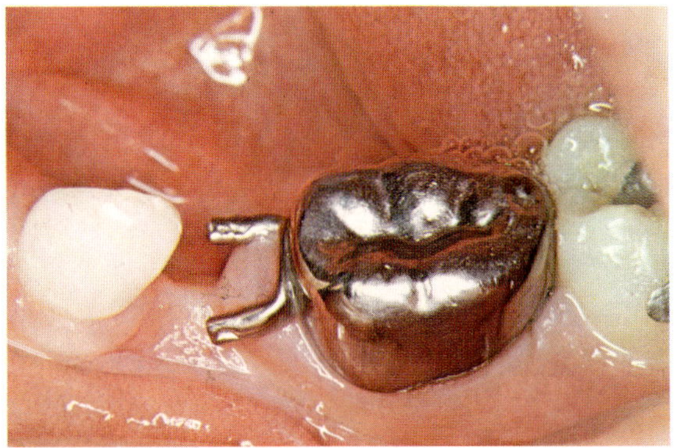

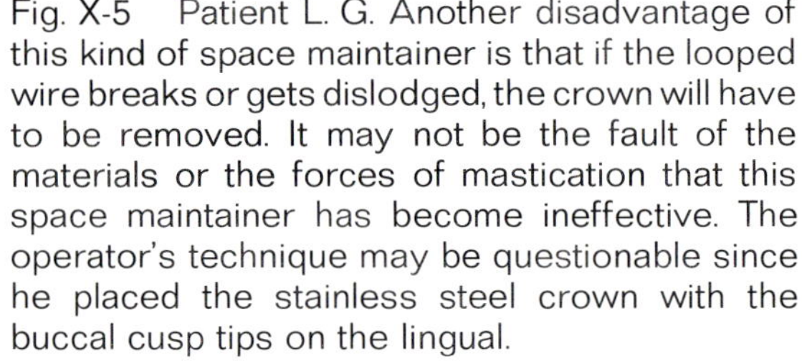

Fig. X-5   Patient L. G. Another disadvantage of this kind of space maintainer is that if the looped wire breaks or gets dislodged, the crown will have to be removed. It may not be the fault of the materials or the forces of mastication that this space maintainer has become ineffective. The operator's technique may be questionable since he placed the stainless steel crown with the buccal cusp tips on the lingual.

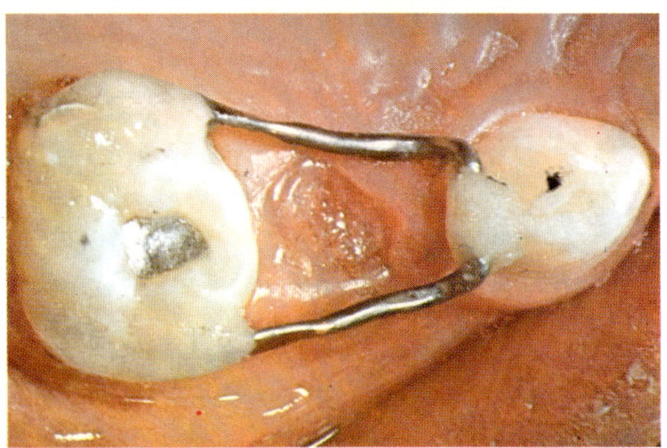

Fig. X-6   Patient A. H. This was one of the first acid etch space maintainers attempted. A pre-formed loop, (Ormco), designed for spot welding on to the bands or stainless steel crowns, was bonded to a deciduous second molar and to a deciduous cuspid.

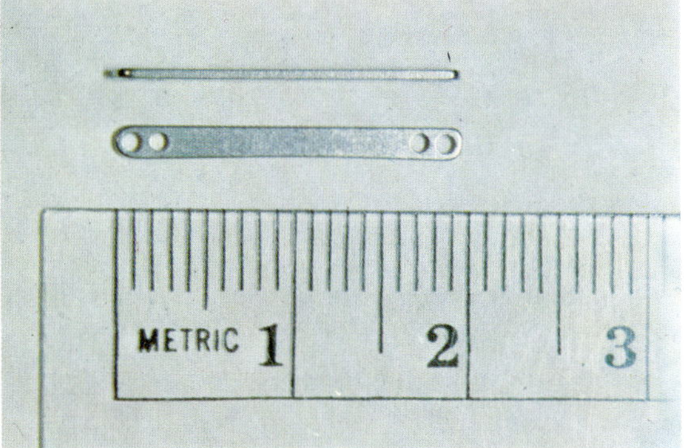

Fig. X-7   Stainless steel bars in this form were ordered for trial use as space maintainers. The ideal length was 2 cm. and each end was perforated with two holes for composite penetration. These space bars have functioned well in two years of clinical trials and are a simple and rapid means of securing space maintenance.

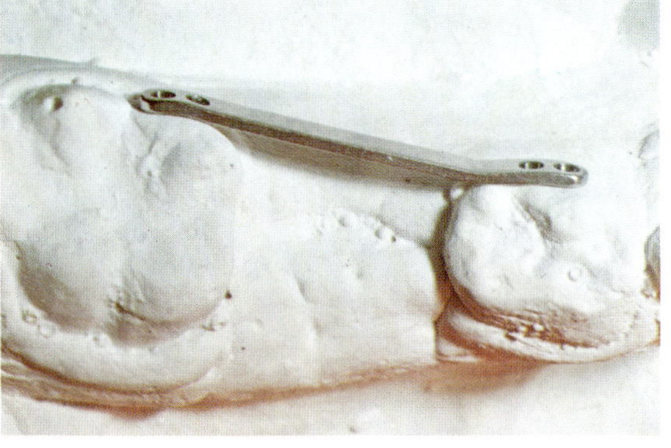

Fig. X-8   Patient M. W. The adaptation of the stainless steel bar can be done in the mouth or on a study model. A three-jawed wire plier is excellent for adapting the bar. The closer the bar can be adapted to the contours of the tooth, the more uniform the thickness of composite will be.

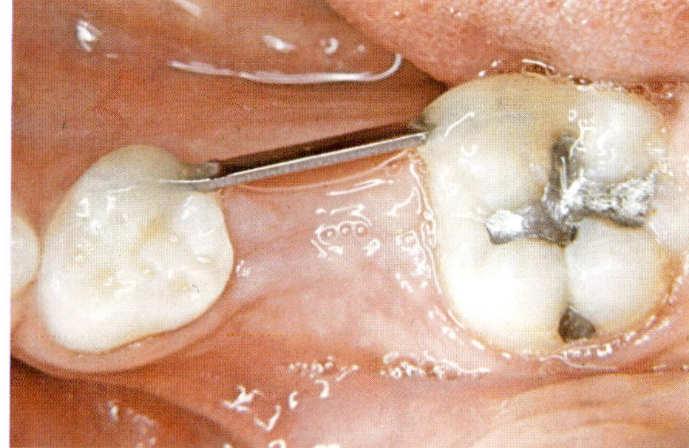

Fig. X-9 Patient M.W. This 6-month recall photograph is of the bar seen in Fig. X-8 (mirror photograph). The composite bond is still in tact and the space maintainer is functioning well. To avoid occlusal interferences it is usually best to bond mandibular space maintainers to the lingual surfaces.

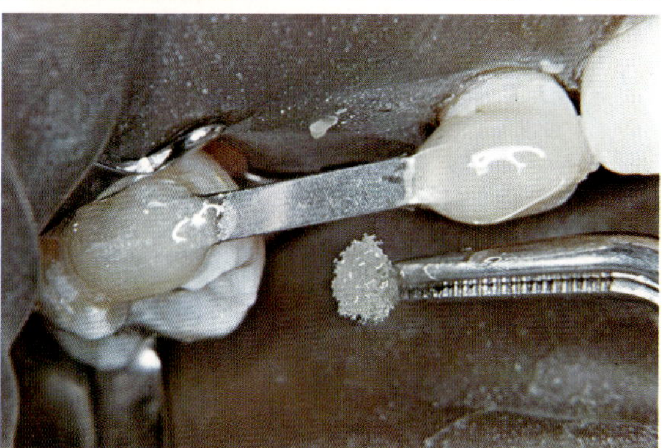

Fig. X-10 Patient G. H. Rubber dam isolation is ideal when bonding space bars. Maxillary space maintainers ideally should be bonded to buccal surfaces to avoid unnecessary grinding for elimination of occlusal interferences. A glaze layer applied to the composite surfaces will give a smooth surface, which is important where composite contacts soft tissue.

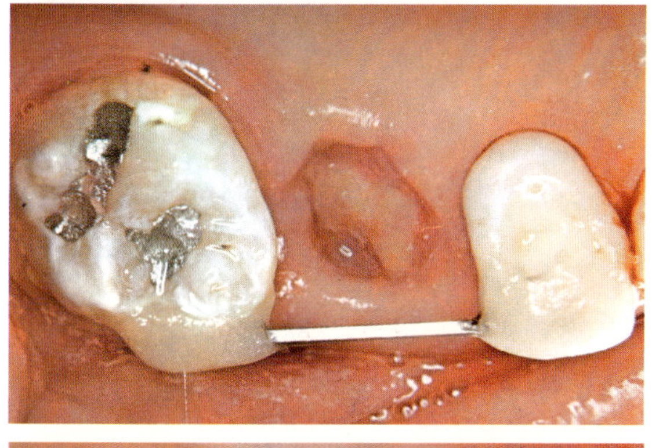

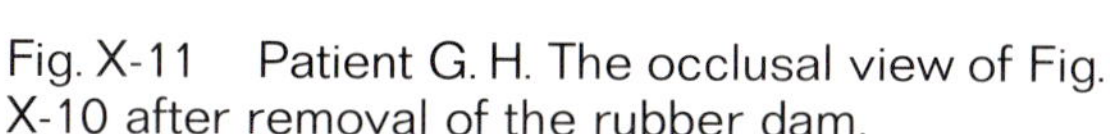

Fig. X-11 Patient G. H. The occlusal view of Fig. X-10 after removal of the rubber dam.

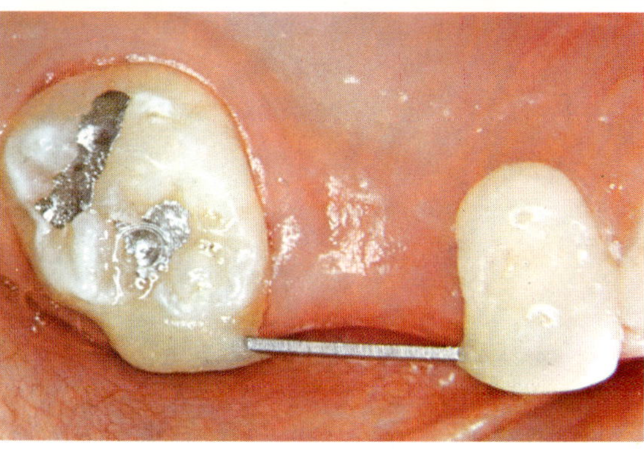

Fig. X-12 Patient G. H. The 12-month recall photograph of Figures X-10 and 11. The bond is firm, the material has worn very little and the space maintainer is performing its function very well with no irritation of soft tissues or predisposition to secondary decay.

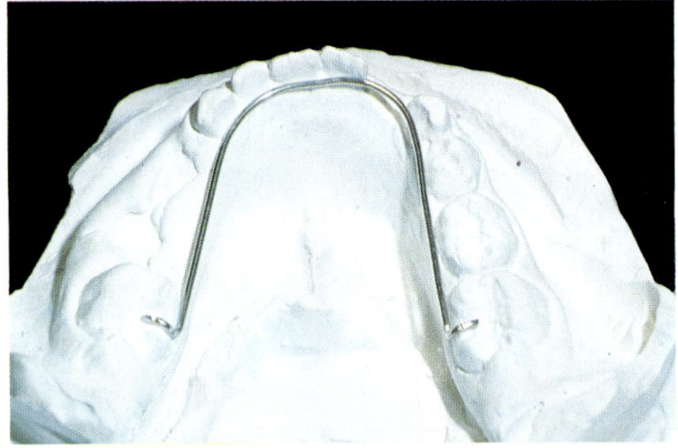

Fig. X-13   Patient M. F. Lingual arch space maintainers can also be bonded to first molars without the use of orthodontic bands. A 0.81 mm (.032″) wire is used and adapted as shown. The wire should contact the lingual surfaces of the anterior teeth, but not any other teeth apart from first permanent molars.

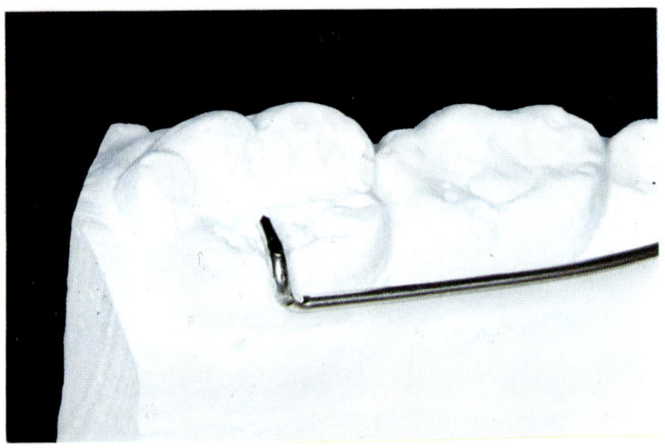

Fig. X-14   Patient G. H. The wire is adapted along the lingual surface of the tooth and then bent into the occlusal groove. This gives added bonding area on the occlusal, in addition to providing further support for the bond to withstand occlusal stresses.

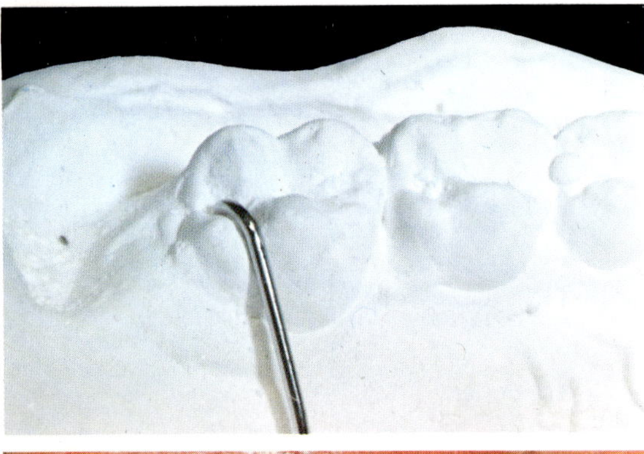

Fig. X-15   Patient F. G. Trans-palatal arches can be equally effectively bonded to first permanent molars. The wire is bent to follow the occluso-lingual groove onto the distal portion of the occlusal surface. This provides adequate bonding area and support against occlusal stress.

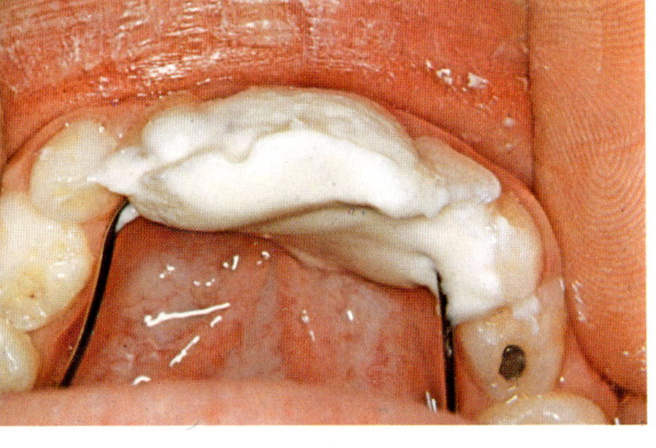

Fig. X-16   Patient G. H. To stabilize the wire in place during bonding, compound impression material or, (as in this case), Alginate, can be used in the anterior region. Alginate placed into the palate will hold a trans-palatal arch in place until bonding is complete.

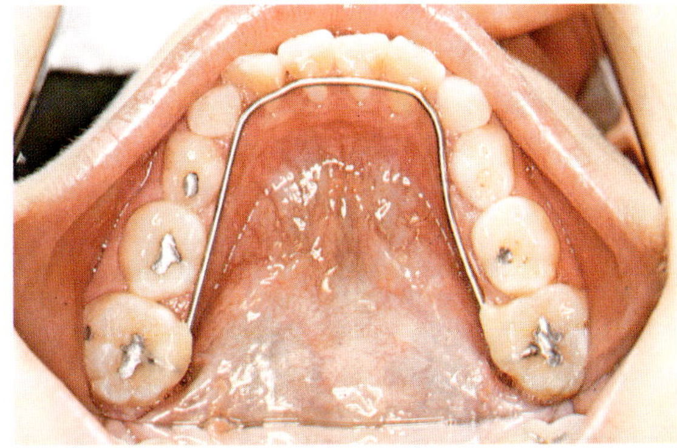

Fig. X-17   Patient G. H. A lingual arch bonded to first permanent molars photographed at the 12-month recall. The arch was placed to prevent tipping of the first permanent molars over ankylosed deciduous molars.

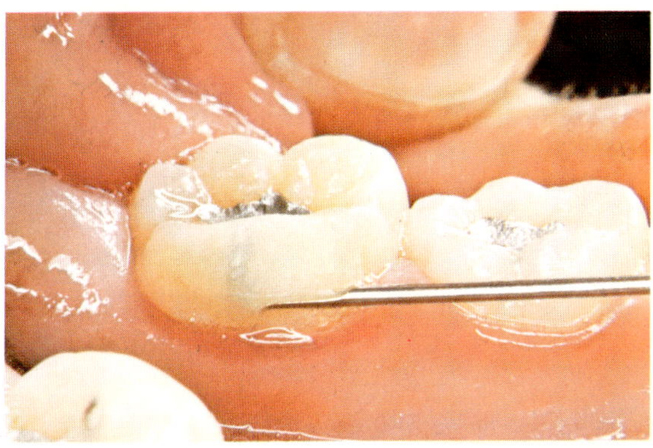

Fig. X-18   Patient G. H. A close-up of the lingual surface bonding area. As frequently happens in these cases, the composite has not bonded well below the wire. It is extremely difficult to apply the composite below the wire without salivary contamination. Composite loss in this case did not affect retention.

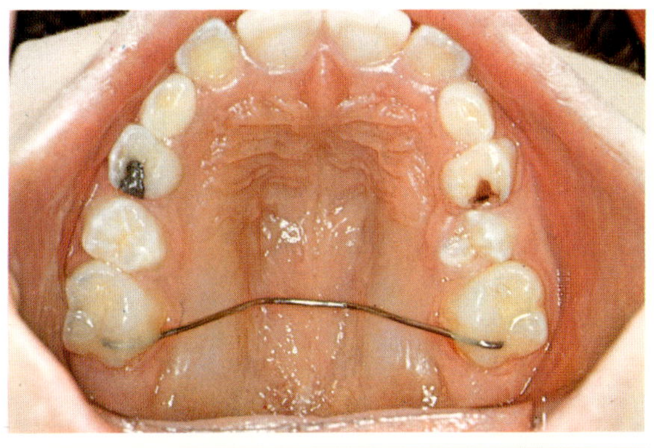

Fig. X-19   Patient F. G. A trans-palatal arch two years after bonding. Despite considerable wear on one of the bonds where the wire shows through the composite, the space maintainer is still functional and shows no sign of detaching. The second bicuspids are erupting and the arch can now be removed after successfully holding the space.

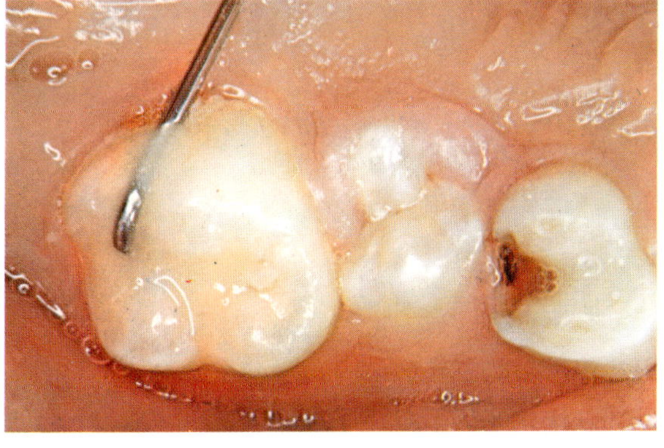

Fig. X-20   Patient F. G. A close-up of the bond showing most wear. Composite was not only applied initially around the wire, but also over the remaining pits and fissures of the occlusal surface to act as a sealant. When removing the wire, the excess composite is trimmed down, leaving enough to cover all grooves for caries protection.

Additional Reading List

Pit and Fissure Sealants:

1. *Bonjanini, J.,* et al.:
Effectiveness of pit and fissure sealants in the prevention of caries. J. of Prev. Dent. 3: 31–34, 1976.

2. *Boudreau, G. E.* and *Jerge, C. R.:*
The efficacy of sealant treatment in the prevention of pit and fissure dental caries: a review and interpretation of literature. JADA 72: 383–387, 1976.

3. *Brooks, J. D.,* et al.:
A comparative study of the retention of two pit and fissure sealants: one-year results. J. of Prev. Dent. 3: 43–46, 1976.

4. *Buonocore, M. G.:*
Adhesive sealing of pits and fissures for caries prevention, with use of ultraviolet light. JADA 80: 324–328, 1970.

5. *Buonocore, M. G.:*
Adhesives for pit and fissures caries control. Dental Clinics of North America 16: 693–708, 1972.

6. *Buonocore, M. G.:*
Caries prevention in pits and fissures sealed with an adhesive resin polymerized by ultraviolet light: a two-year study of a single adhesive application. JADA 82: 1090–1093, 1971.

7. *Buonocore, M. G.:*
Sealants: Questions and answers. JASPD, 1973.

8. *Burt, B. A., Berman, D. S.,* and *Silverstone, L. M.:*
Sealant retention and effects on occlusal caries after 2 years in a public program. Community Dent. Oral Epidemiol. 5: 15–21, 1977.

9. *Charbeneau, G. T., Dennison, J. B.,* and *Ryge, G.:*
A filled pit and fissure sealant: 18-month results. JADA 95: 299–306, 1977.

10. *Chow, L. C.* and *Brown, W. E.:*
Topical fluoridation of teeth before sealant application. J. Dent. Res. 54: 1089, 1975.

11. *Cons, N. C., Pollard, S. T.,* and *Leske, G. S.:*
Adhesive sealant clinical trial: results of a three-year study in a fluoridated area. J. Prev. Dent. 3, 3: 14–19, 1976.

12. *Cueto, E. I.* and *Buonocore, M. G.:*
Sealing of pits and fissures with an adhesive resin: its use in caries prevention. JADA 75: 121–128, 1967.

13. *Eames, W. B.:*
Pit & fissure sealants. 1972.

14. *Ferrara, C. M.:*
Pit and fissure sealants. NYSDJ 41: 536–543, 1975.

15. *Fan, P. L., Seluk, L. W.,* and *O'Brian, W. J.:*
Penetravity of sealants. I. J. Dent Res. 54: 262–264, 1975.

16. *Going, R. E.,* et al.:
Two-year clinical evaluation of a pit and fissure sealant. Part I: Retention and loss of substance. JADA 92: 388–397, 1976.

17. *Going, R. E.,* et al.:
Two-year clinical evaluation of a pit and fissure sealant. Part II: Caries initiation and progression. JADA 92: 578–585, 1976.

18. *Going, R. E.,* et al.:
Four-year clinical evalutation of a pit and fissure sealant. JADA 95: 972–981, 1977.

19. *Gourley, J. M.:*
A two-year study of a fissure sealant in two Nova Scotia communities. J. Public Health Dent. 35: 132–137, 1975.

20. *Gwinnett, A. J.* and *Buonocore, M. G.:*
Adhesives and caries prevention. British Dental Journal, 1965.

21. *Gwinnett, A. J.:*
Caries prevention through sealing of pits and fissures. J. of Canadian Dent. Assoc. 37, 1971.

22. *Gwinnett, A. J.:*
The bonding of sealants to enamel. JASPD pp. 21–29, February, 1973.

23. *Gwinnett, A. J.:*
The scientific basis of the sealant procedure. J. Prev. Dent. 3, 2: 15–28, 1976.

24. *Handelman, S. L., Buonocore, M. G., and Heseck, D. J.:*
A preliminary report on the effect of fissure sealant on bacteria in dental caries. J. Prosthet. Dent. 27: 390–392, 1972.

25. *Handelman, S. L., Buonocore, M. G., and Schoute, P. C.:*
Progress report on the effect of a fissure sealant on bacteria in dental caries. JADA 87: 1189–1191, 1973.

26. *Handelman, S. L.:*
Microbiologic aspects of sealing carious lesions. J. Prev. Dent. 3, 2: 29–32, 1976.

27. *Handelman, S. L., Washburn, F., and Wopperer, P.:*
Two-year report of sealant effect on bacteria in dental caries. JADA 93: 967–970, 1976.

28. *Harris, N. O., et al.:*
Adhesive sealant clinical trial: effectiveness in a school population of the U.S. Virgin Islands. J. Prev. Dent. 3, 3: 27–37, 1976.

29. *Hinding, J. H. and Buonocore, M. G.:*
The effects of varying the application protocol on the retention of pit and fissure sealant: a two-year study. JADA 89: 127–131, 1974.

30. *Horowitz, H. S., Heifetz, S. B., and McCune, R. J.:*
The effectiveness of an adhesive sealant in preventing occlusal caries: findings after two years in Kalispell, Montana. JADA 89: 885–890, 1974.

31. *Horowitz, H. S., Heifetz, S. B., and Poulsen, S.:*
Adhesive sealant clinical trial: an overview of results after four years in Kalispell, Montana. J. Prev. Dent. 3, 3: 38–49, 1976.

32. *Horowitz, H. S., Heifetz, S. B., and Poulsen, S.:*
Retention and effectiveness of an adhesive sealant after five years. AADR abstract no. 72, J. Dent. Res., June 1977.

33. *Ibsen, R. L.:*
Use of a filled diacrylate as fissure sealant: one-year clinical study. JASPD 3: 60–65, 1973.

34. *Kopel, H. M. and Grenoble, D. E.:*
The pit and fissure sealants: A critical review. J. Southern Cal. Dent. Assn. 41: 103–109, 1973.

35. *Lee, H. L. and Swartz, M. L.:*
Sealing of Developmental Pits and Fissures: I. In Vitro Study. J. Dent. Res., January 1971.

36. *Lee, H. L., et al.:*
Sealing of Developmental Pits and Fissures: III. Effects of Fluoride on Adhesion of Rigid and Flexible Sealers. J. Dent. Res. 51: 191–201, 1972.

37. *Lee, H. and Ocumpaugh, D.:*
Sealing of developmental pits and fissures. V. Comparison of adhesive topical fluoride coating vs. Fluoride gels. Biomat., Med. Dev. Art. Org., 1 (1), 163–170, 1973.

38. *Leske, G. S., Pollard, S., and Cons, N.:*
The effectiveness of dental hygienist teams in applying pit and fissure sealants. J. Prev. Dent. 3, 2: 33–36, 1976.

39. *Low, T., von Fraunhofer, J. A., and Winter, G. B.:*
Influence of the topical application of fluoride on the in vitro adhesion of fissure sealants. J. Dent. Res. 56: 17–20, 1977.

40. *Lund, M. R.:*
Treatment of grooves with sealants utilizing acid etching. Indiana Dent. Assn. J. pp. 15–17, January 1974.

41. *McCune, R. J., et al.:*
Pit and fissure sealants: one-year results from a study in Kalispell, Montana. JADA 87: 1177–1180, 1973.

42. *McLean, J. W. and Wilson, A. D.:*
Fissure sealing and filling with an adhesive glass-ionomer cement. Brit. Dent. J. 136: 269–276, 1974.

43. *Pahlavan, A., Dennison, J. B., and Charbeneau, G. T.:*
Penetration of restorative resins into acid-etched human enamel. JADA 93: 1170–1176, 1976.

44. *Powell, P. B., et al.:*
Microleakage around a pit and fissure sealant. J. of Dent. for Child. pp. 18–21, 1977.

45. *Ripa, L. W. and Cole, W. W.:*
Occlusal sealing and caries prevention: Results 12 months after a single application of adhesive resin. J. Dent. Res. pp. 171–173, January 1970.

46. *Ripa, L. W.:*
Occlusal Sealing: Rationale of the technique and historical review. JASPD, pp. 32–39, January 1973.

47. *Ripa, L. W.:*
The current status of occlusal sealants. J. Prev. Dent. 3, 2: 6–14, 1976.

48. *Rock, W. P.:*
Fissure sealants: Results obtained with two different sealants after one year. Brit. Dent. J., pp. 146–151, 1972.

49. *Rock, W. P.:*
Fissure sealants: further results of clinical trials. Brit. Dent. J., pp. 317–321, 1974.

50. *Rock, W. P.:*
The use of ultra-violet radiation in dentistry. Brit. Dent. J., pp. 455–458, 1974.

51. *Rock, W. P.:*
The effect of etching of human enamel upon bond strengths with fissure sealant resins. Arch. Oral Biol. 19: 873–877, 1974.

52. *Rock, W. P.:*
Fissure sealants: Results of a 3-year clinical trial using an ultra-violet sensitive resin. Brit. Dent. J., pp. 16–18, 1977.

53. *Roydhouse, R. H.:*
Prevention of occlusal fissure caries by use of a sealant: A pilot study. J. of Dent. for Child., 253–262, May 1968.

54. *Ryge, G.* and *Baskin, P.:*
The future of pit and fissure sealants. JASPD, 54–57, January 1973.

55. *Sheykholeslam, Z.* and *Buonocore, M. G.:*
Bonding of resins to phosphoric acid-etched enamel surfaces of permanent and deciduous teeth. J. Dent. Res. 51: 1572–1576, 1972.

56. *Sheykholeslam, Z., Buonocore, M. G.,* and *Gwinnett, A. J.:*
Effect of fluorides on the bonding of resins to phosphoric acid-etched bovine enamel. Arch. Oral Biol. 17: 1037–1045, 1972.

57. *Silverstone, L. M.:*
Fissure sealants. Caries Res. 8: 2–26, 1974.

58. *Silverstone, L. M.:*
Should I be using pit and fissure sealants or amalgam? Int. Dent. J. 26: 29–40, March 1976.

59. *Simonsen, R. J.* and *Stallard, R. E.:*
Fissure sealants: Colored sealant retention 3 months post application. Quintessence Int. 8: 1–6, 1977.

60. *Simonsen, R. J.* and *Stallard, R. E.:*
Sealant-restorations utilizing a diluted filled composite resin: one year results. Quintessence Int. 6: 77–84, 1977.

61. *Stiles, H. M.,* et al.:
Adhesive sealant clinical trial: Comparative results of application by a dentist or dental auxiliaries. J. Prev. Dent. 3, 3: 8–13, 1976.

62. *Sveen, O. B.* and *Hinding, J. H.:*
Sealants—A milestone in preventive dentistry? JADA, pp. 401–406, November 1971.

63. *Swartz, M. L.,* et al.:
Addition of fluoride to pit and fissure sealants—A feasibility study. J. Dent. Res. 55: 757–771, 1976.

64. *Taylor, C. L.* and *Gwinnett, A. J.:*
A study of the penetration of sealants into pits and fissures. JADA 87: 1181–1188, 1973.

65. *Ulvestad, H.:*
Clinical trials with fissure sealant materials in Scandinavia. Proceedings of an International Symposium on the Acid Etch Technique. *Silverstone, L. M.* and *Dogon, I. L.* (Eds.). North Central Publishing Co., St. Paul, Minnesota, pp. 165–175, 1975.

66. *Ulvestad, H.:*
A 24-month evaluation of fissure sealing with a diluted composite material. Scand. J. Dent. Res. 84: 51–55, 1976.

67. *Ulvestad, H.:*
Evaluation of fissure sealing with a diluted composite sealant and an UV-light polymerized sealant after 36 months' observation. Scand. J. Dent. Res. 84: 401–403, 1976.

68. *Whitehurst, V. W.* and *Soni, N. N.:*
Adhesive sealant clinical trial: results eighteen months after one application. J. Prev. Dent. 3, 3: 20–26, 1976.

69. *Williams, B.* and *Winter, G. B.:*
Fissure sealants: A 2-year clinical trial. Brit. Dent. J., pp. 15–18, July 1976.

70. *Wilkins, J. S.* and *Phillips, R. W.:*
Testing of pit and fissure sealants in the monkey. J. Prosthet. Dent., pp. 666–673, 1977.

71. *Woody, R. D., Moffa, J. P.* and *McCune, R. J.:*
Assessment of leakage of four pit and fissure sealant materials by Ca[45]. IADR abstract no. 717, 1972.

72. *Yankelson, M.:*
The acid etch in orthodontics: the problem. Proceedings of an International Symposium on the Acid Etch Technique. Silverstone, L. M., Dogon, I. L. (Eds.). North Central Publishing Co., St. Paul, Minnesota, pp. 255–264, 1975.

Resin:

73. *Antonucci, J. M.* and *Bowen, R. L.:*
Dimethacrylates derived from hydroxybenzoic acids. J. Dent. Res. 55: 8–15, 1976.

74. *Argentar, H.* and *Bowen, R. L.:*
Colored charge-transfer complexes from N,N-dimethyl-p-toluidine. J. Dent. Res. 54: 588–598, 1975.

75. *Bailey, A. R., Shovelton, D. S.,* and *Wilson, H. J.:*
A new composite restorative material. Brit. Dent. J. pp. 311–317, 1973.

76. *Barton, J. A., Jr.,* et al.:
An experimental radiopaque composite material, J. Dent. Res. 52: 731–739, 1973.

77. *Bowen, R. L.:*
Use of epoxy resins in restorative materials. J. Dent. Res. 35: 360–369, 1956.

78. *Bowen, R. L.:*
Investigation of the surface of hard tooth tissues by a surface activity test. *Phillips, R. W. and Ryge, G.* (Eds.): Proceedings of the workshop on adhesive restorative dental materials at Indiana University, Sept. 28–29, 1961, Spencer Indiana: Owen Litho Service, pp. 177–191.

79. *Bowen, R. L. and Rodriguez, M. S.:*
Tensile strength and modulus of elasticity of tooth structure and several restorative materials. JADA 64: 378–387, 1962.

80. *Bowen, R. L.:*
Dental filling material comprising vinyl silane treated fused silica and a binder consisting of the reaction product of Bisphenol and glycidyl acrylate, Washington, DC: Commissioner of Patents & Trademarks, US Patent No. 3,066,112, Nov. 1962.

81. *Bowen, R. L.:*
Properties of a silica-reinforced polymer for dental restorations. JADA 66: 57–64, 1963.

82. *Bowen, R. L.:*
Effect of particle shape and size distribution in a reinforced polymer. JADA 69: 481–495, 1964.

83. *Bowen, R. L.:*
Method of preparing a monomer having phenoxy and methacrylate groups linked by hydroxy glycerol groups, Washington, DC: Commissioner of Patents & Trademarks, US Patent No. 3,179,623, April 1965.

84. *Bowen, R. L.:*
Silica-resin direct filling material and method of preparation, Washington, DC: Commissioner of Patents & Trademarks, US Patent No. 3,194,783, July 1965.

85. *Bowen, R. L.:*
Silica-resin direct filling material and method of preparation, Washington, DC: Commissioner of Patents & Trademarks, US Patent No. 3,194,784, July 1965.

86. *Bowen, R. L.:*
Surface-active comonomer and method of preparation, Washington, DC: Commissioner of Patents & Trademarks, US Patent No. 3,200,142, August 1965.

87. *Bowen, R. L.:*
Adhesive bonding of various materials to hard tooth tissues: I. Method of determining bond strength. J. Dent. Res. 44: 690–95, 1965.

88. *Bowen, R. L.:*
Adhesive bonding of various materials to hard tooth tissues: II. Bonding to dentin promoted by a surface-active comonomer. J. Dent. Res. 44: 895–902, 1965.

89. *Bowen, R. L.:*
Adhesive bonding of various materials to hard tooth tissues: III. Bonding to dentin improved by pretreatment and the use of a surface-active comonomer. J. Dent. Res. 44: 903–905, 1965.

90. *Bowen, R. L.:*
Adhesive bonding of various materials to hard tooth tissues: IV. Bonding to dentin, enamel, and fluorapatite improved by the use of a surface-active comonomer. J. Dent. Res. 44: 906–911, 1965.

91. *Bowen, R. L.:*
Adhesive bonding of various materials to hard tooth tissues: V. The effect of a surface-active comonomer on adhesion to diverse substrates. J. Dent. Res. 44: 1369–1373, 1965.

92. *Bowen, R. L.:*
Adhesive bonding of various materials to hard tooth tissues: VI. Forces developing in direct filling materials during hardening. JADA 74: 439–445, 1967.

93. *Bowen, R. L.:*
Development of an adhesive restorative material, in adhesive restorative dental materials II, University of Virginia Workshop, Public Health Service Publication No. 1494, Washington, DC: US Gov. Printing Office, 1966, pp. 225–231.

94. *Bowen, R. L. and Argentar, H.:*
Diminishing discoloration in methacrylate accelerator systems. JADA 75: 918–923, 1967.

95. *Bowen, R. L., Paffenbarger, G. C. and Mullineaux, A. L.:*
A laboratory and clinical comparison of silicate cements and a direct-filling resin: A progress report. J. Pros. Dent. 20: 426–437, 1968.

96. *Bowen, R. L. and Cleek, G. W.:*
X-ray-opaque reinforcing fillers for composite materials. J. Dent. Res. 48: 79–82, 1969.

97. *Bowen, R. L. and Mullineaux, A. L.:*
Adhesive restorative materials, Dent. Abstracts 14: 80–82, 1969.

98. *Bowen, R. L.:*
Adhesion-promoting materials, Washington, DC: Commissioner of Patents & Trademarks, US Patent No. 3,635,889, Jan. 18, 1972.

99. *Bowen, R. L.:*
Crystalline dimethacrylate monomers. J. Dent. Res. 49: 810–815, 1970.

100. *Bowen, R. L. and Argentar, H.:*
Amine accelerators for methacrylate resin systems. J. Dent. Res. 50: 923–928, 1971.

101. *Bowen, R. L. and Argentar, H.:*
Tertiary aromatic amine accelerators with molecular weights above 400. J. Dent. Res. 51: 473–482, 1972.

102. *Bowen, R. L.* and *Cleek, G. W.:*
A new series of X-ray-opaque reinforcing fillers for composite materials. J. Dent. Res. 51: 177–182, 1972.

103. *Bowen, R. L.:*
Tertiary eutectic dimethacrylate monomer system and restorative dental material prepared therefrom, Washington, DC: Commissioner of Patents & Trademarks, US Patent No. 3,539,526, 1970.

104. *Bowen, R.L., Barton, J.A., Jr.,* and *Mullineaux, A.L.:*
Composite restorative materials, in *Dickinson, G. R.,* and *Cassel, J. M.* (Eds.): Dental Materials Research, Washington, DC: National Bureau of Standards, Special Publication 354, US Government Printing Office, 1972, pp. 93–100.

105. *Bowen, R. L.* and *Argentar, H.:*
Tertiary aromatic amine accelerators in dental compositions, Washington, DC: Commissioner of Patents & Trademarks, US Patent No. 3,740,850, 1973.

106. *Bowen, R. L.* and *Argentar, H.:*
A stabilizing comonomer: I. Synthesis and confirmation of structure. J. Dent. Res. 51: 1071–1074, 1972.

107. *Bowen, R. L.* and *Argentar, H.:*
A stabilizing comonomer: II. Stabilization and polymerization characteristics. J. Dent. Res. 51: 1614–1618, 1972.

108. *Bowen, R. L.* and *Chandler, H. H.:*
Metal-filled resin composites, J. Dent. Res. 52: 522–532, 1973.

109. *Bowen, R. L.* and *Argentar, H.:*
A method for determining the optimum peroxide-to-amine ratio for self-curing resins. J. Applied Polymer Sci. 17: 2213–2222, 1973.

110. *Bowen, R. L.:*
Dental primer varnish, Washington, DC: Commissioner of Patents & Trademarks, US Patent No. 3,785,832, Jan. 15, 1974.

111. *Bowen, R. L.* and *Antonucci, J. M.:*
Dimethylacrylate monomers of aromatic diethers. J. Dent. Res. 54: 599–604, 1975.

112. *Bowen, R. L., Chandler, H. H.* and *Wyckoff, H. O.:*
Additional studies of metal-filled resin composites. (Manuscript submitted for publication.)

113. *Bowen, R. L.:*
Adhesive bonding of various materials to hard tooth tissues: VII. Metal salts as mordants for coupling agents, in *Moskowitz, H. D., Ward, G. T.* and *Woolridge, F. D.* (Eds.): Dental adhesive materials, Proceedings from Symposium held Nov. 8–9, 1973 at the Hunter-Bellevue School of Nursing, New York City: Prestige Graphic Services 1974, pp. 205–221.

114. *Bowen, R. L.:*
Adhesive bonding of various materials to hard tooth tissues: IX. The concept of polyfunctional surface-active comonomers, presented at the 7th National Bureau of Standards in-Action Seminar "Health Related Activities": Gaithersburg, Maryland, Dec. 14, 1973, J. Biomed. Mater Res. No. 5: 501–510, 1975.

115. *Bowen, R. L.* and *Reed, L. E.:*
Semiporous reinforcing fillers for composite resins: I. Preparation of provisional glass formulations. J. Dent. Res. 55: 738–747, 1976.

116. *Bowen, R. L.* and *Reed, L. E.:*
Semiporous reinforcing fillers for composite resins: II. Heat treatment and etching characteristics. J. Dent. Res. 55: 748–756, 1976.

117. *Buonocore, M.G., Wileman, W.,* and *Brudevold, F.:*
A report on a resin composition capable of bonding to human dentin surfaces. J. Dent. Res. 35: 846–851, 1956.

118. *Buonocore, M. G.* and *Quigley, J.:*
Bonding of synthetic resin material to human dentin: preliminary histological study of the bond area. JADA 57: 807, 1958.

119. *Buonocore, M. G.:*
Principles of adhesive retention and adhesive restorative materials. JADA 67: 382–391, 1963.

120. *Buonocore, M. G.* and *Casciani, C.:*
Synthesis and properties of certain urethanes of potential use in restorative dentistry—a preliminary report. NYSDJ 35: 135–147, 1969.

121. *Chandler, H. H.,* et al.:
Clinical investigation of a radiopaque composite restorative material. JADA 50: 935–940, 1971.

122. *Chandler, H. H., Bowen, R. L.,* and *Paffenbarger, G. C.:*
The need for radiopaque denture base materials. A review of the literature. J. Biomed. Mat. Res. 5: 245–252, 1971.

123. *Chandler, H. H., Bowen, R. L.,* and *Paffenbarger, G. C.:*
Development of a radiopaque denture base material. J. Biomed. Mat. Res. 5: 253–265, 1971.

124. *Chandler, H. H., Bowen, R. L.,* and *Paffenbarger, G. C.:*
Physical properties of a radiopaque denture base material. J. Biomed. Mat. Res. 5: 335–357, 1971.

125. *Chandler, H. H., Bowen, R. L.,* and *Paffenbarger, G. C.:*
Radiopaque denture base materials: Technic Dentures. J. Biomed. Mat. Res. 5: 359–371, 1971.

126. *Chandler, H. H., Bowen, R. L., and Paffenbarger, G. C.:*
A method for finishing composite restorative materials. JADA 83: 344–348, 1971.

127. *Chandler, H. H., et al.:*
Clinical evaluation of a radiopaque composite restorative material after three and one half years. J. Dent. Res. 52: 1128–1137, 1973.

128. *Chandler, H. H. et al.:*
Clinical evaluation of a tooth-restoration coupling agent. JADA 88: 114–118, 1974.

129. *Eames, W. B., O'Neal, S. J., and Rogers, L. B.:*
Composite plain talk. JADA 92: 550–554, 1976.

130. *Eames, W. B., O'Neal, S. J., and Monteiro, J.:*
Resin Veneers. Product Report.

131. *Eden, G. T., Craig, R. G., and Peyton, F. A.:*
Evaluation of a tensile test for direct filling resins. J. Dent. Res. 49: 428–434, 1970.

132. *Eliasson, S. T., et al.:*
Surface problems with composite resin restorations. Northwest Dentistry 55: 70–74, 1976.

133. *Eriksen, H. M. and Buonocore, M. G.:*
Marginal leakage with different composite restorative materials: effect of restorative techniques. JADA 93: 1143–1148, 1976.

134. *Galligan, J. D., Schwartz, A. M., and Minor, F. W.:*
Adhesive polyurethane liners for anterior restorations. J. Dent. Res. 74: 629–632, 1968.

135. *Kusy, R. P. and Leinfelder, K. F.:*
Pattern of wear in posterior composite restorations. J. Dent. Res. 56: 544, 1977.

136. *Lee, H.:*
Adhesions between living tissue and plastics. I. Adhesion of epoxy and polyurethane resins to dentin and enamel. J. Biomed. Mat. Res. 3: 349, 1969.

137. *Lee, H. L., Jr. and Swartz, M. L.:*
Scanning electron microscope study of composite restorative materials. J. Dent. Res. 49: 149–158, 1970.

138. *Lee, H. L., et al.:*
An adhesive dental restorative material. J. Dent. Res. 50: 125–132, 1971.

139. *Lee, H. L., Orlowski, J. A., and Rogers, B. J.:*
A comparison of ultraviolet-curing and self-curing polymers in preventive, restorative and orthodontic dentistry. Inter. Dental J. 26: 134–151, 1976.

140. *McLundie, A. C. and Murray, F. D.:*
Silicate cements and composite resins—A scanning electron microscope study. J. Prosthet. Dent. 27: 544–551, 1972.

141. *Misra, D. N., Bowen, R. L., and Wallace, B. M.:*
Adhesive bonding of various materials to hard tooth tissues: VIII. Nickel and copper ions on hydroxyapatite; role of ion exchange and surface nucleation, J. Coll. & Interface Sci. 51 No. 1: 36–43, 1975.

142. *Misra, D. N. and Bowen, R. L.:*
Adhesive bonding of various materials to hard tooth tissues: XI. Chemisorption of the adduct of diglycidyl ether of bisphenol A with N-phenylglycine on hydroxylapathite, J. Phys. Chem. 81: No. 9: 842–846, 1977.

143. *Misra, D. N. and Bowen, R. L.:*
Sorption of water by filled resin composites. J. Dent. Res. 56: 603–612, 1977.

144. *Paffenbarger, G. C., Sweeney, W. T., and Bowen, R. L.:*
Bonding porcelain teeth to acrylic resin denture base, JADA 74: 1018–1023, 1967.

145. *Pameijer, C. H. and Stallard, R. E.:*
The fallacy of polishing composite restorations. J. of Dent. Prac. 1973.

146. *Peterson, E. A., Phillips, R. W., and Swartz, M. L.:*
A comparison of the physical properties of four restorative resins. JADA 73: 1324–1336, 1966.

147. *Phillips, R. W.:*
Advancements in adhesive restorative dental materials. J. Dent. Res. 45: 1662–1667, 1966.

148. *Pugnier, V. A. and Jordan, W. A.:*
The role of cyanoacrylate resins in caries prevention. Northwest Dentistry, pp. 177–179, 1971.

149. *Pugnier, V. A.:*
Cyanoacrylate resins in caries prevention: a two-year study. JADA 84: 829–831, 1972.

150. *Rider, M., Tanner, A. N., and Kenny, B.:*
Investigation of adhesive properties of dental composite materials using an improved tensile test procedure and scanning electron microscopy. J. Dent. Res. 56: 368–378, 1977.

151. *Rose, E. E., et al.:*
The screening of materials for adhesion to human tooth structure. J. Dent. Res. 34: 577–586, 1955.

152. *Rupp, N. W., Bowen, R. L., and Paffenbarger, G. C.:*
Bonding cold-curing denture base acrylic resin to acrylic resin teeth. JADA 83: 601–606, 1971.

153. *Schouboe, P. J., Paffenbarger, G. C., and Sweeney, W. T.:*
Resin cements and posterior-type direct filling resins. JADA 52: 584–600, 1956.

Anterior Fracture Restoration:

154. *Buonocore, M. G. and Davile, J.:*
Restoration of fractured anterior teeth with ultraviolet light polymerized bonding materials, a new technique. JADA 86: 1349–1354, 1973.

155. *Flynn, M.:*
Clinical evaluation of two pinless incisal edge repairs: a 24-month study. JADA 94: 97–99, 1977.

156. *Jordan, R. E.,* et al.:
Restoration of fractured and hypoplastic incisors by the acid etch resin technique: a three-year report. JADA 95: 795–803, 1977.

157. *Meurman, J. H.* and *Helminen, S. K. J.:*
Repair of fractured incisal edges with ultraviolet-light activated fissure sealant and composite resin. Proc. Finn. Dent. Soc. 70: 186–190, 1974.

158. *Roberts, M. W.* and *Moffa, J. P.:*
Restoration of fractured incisal angles with an ultraviolet activated sealant and a composite resin—a case report. J. of Dent. for Child., Sept. 1972.

Enamel:

159. *Albert, N.* and *Grenoble, D. E.:*
An in vivo study of enamel remineralization after acid etching. JSCDA 39: 747–751, 1971.

160. *Bozalis, W. G.* and *Marshall, G. W.:*
Acid etching patterns of primary enamel. J. Dent. Res. 56: 185, 1977.

161. *Brauer, B. M.* and *Termini, D. J.:*
Bonding of bovine enamel to restorative resin: effect of pretreatment of enamel. J. Dent. Res. 51: 151–159, 1972.

162. *Buonocore, M. G., Matsui, A.,* and *Gwinnett, A. J.:*
Penetration of resin dental materials into enamel surfaces with reference to bonding. Arch. Oral Biol. 13: 61–70, 1968.

163. *Conniff, J. N.* and *Hamby, G. R.:*
Preparation of primary tooth enamel for acid conditioning. J. of Dent. for Child., May–June 1976.

164. *Cooley, W. E.:*
Reactions of tin (II) and fluoride ions with etched enamel. J. Dent. Res. 40: 1199–1210, 1961.

165. *Darling, A. I.:*
Resistance of the enamel to dental caries. J. Dent. Res. 42: 488–496, 1963.

166. *Eidelman, E.:*
The structure of the enamel in primary teeth: practical applications in restorative techniques. J. of Dent. for Child., May–June 1976.

167. *Frank, R. M.* and *Brendel, A.:*
Ultrastructure of the approximal dental plaque and the underlying normal and carious enamel. Arch. Oral Biol. 11: 883–912, 1966.

168. *Fremlin, J. H., Mathieson, J.,* and *Hardwick, J. L.:*
The preparation of thin sections of dental enamel. Arch. Oral Biol. 5: 55–60, 1961.

169. *Gillings, B.* and *Buonocore, M. G.:*
Thickness of enamel at the base of pits and fissures in human molars and bicuspids. J. Dent. Res. 40: 119–133, 1961.

170. *Goland, P., Scheiman-Tagger, E.,* and *Engel, M.:*
Enamel preservation during decalcification following fixation by some reactive halogen compounds. J. Dent. Res. 44: 342–349, 1965.

171. *Gray, J. A.:*
Kinetics of enamel dissolution during formation of incipient caries-like lesions. Arch. Oral Biol. 11: 397–421, 1966.

172. *Gwinnett, A. J.:*
The ultrastructure of the "prismless" enamel of deciduous teeth. Arch. Oral Biol. 11: 1109–1115, 1966.

173. *Gwinnett, A. J.:*
The ultrastructure of the "prismless" enamel of permanent human teeth. Arch. Oral Biol. 12: 381–387, 1967.

174. *Gwinnett, A. J.:*
A study of enamel adhesives: The physical relationship between enamel and adhesive. Arch. Oral Biol. 12: 1615–1620, 1967.

175. *Gwinnett, A. J.:*
Morphology of the interface between adhesive resins and treated human enamel fissures as seen by scanning electron microscopy. Arch. Oral Biol. 16: 237–238, 1971.

176. *Gwinnett, A. J.:*
Histologic changes in human enamel following treatment with acidic adhesive conditioning agents. Arch. Oral Biol. 16: 731–738, 1971.

177. *Gwinnett, A. J., Buonocore, M. G.,* and *Skeykholeslam, Z.:*
Effect of fluoride on etched human and bovine tooth enamel surfaces as demonstrated by scanning electron microscopy. Archs. Oral Biol. 17: 271–278, 1972.

178. *Gwinnett, A. J.* and *Buonocore, M. G.:*
A scanning electron microscope study of pit and fissure surfaces conditioned for adhesive sealing. Arch. Oral Biol. 17: 415–423, 1972.

179. *Gwinnett, A. J.* and *Ripa, L. W.:*
Penetration of pit and fissure sealants into conditioned human enamel. Arch. Oral Biol. 18: 435–439, 1973.

180. *Gwinnett. A. J.:*
The sequence of topical fluoride and occlusal sealant applications, JASPD, pp. 54–57, 1973.

181. *Gwinnett, A. J.:*
Human prismless enamel and its influence on sealant penetration. Arch Oral Biol. 18: 441–444, 1973.

182. *Gwinnett, A. J.:*
Structural changes in enamel and dentin of fractured anterior teeth after acid conditioning. JADA 86: 117–122, 1973.

183. *Hinding, J. H. and Sveen, O. B.:*
A scanning electron microscope study of the effects of acid conditioning on the occlusal enamel of human permanent and deciduous teeth. Arch. Oral Biol. 19: 573–576, 1974.

184. *Hinrichsen, C. F. L. and Engel, M. B.:*
Fine structure of partially demineralized enamel. Arch. Oral Biol. 11: 65–93, 1966.

185. *Hoffman, S., McEwan, W. S., and Drew, C. M.:*
Scanning electron microscope studies of dental enamel. J. Dent. Res. 48: 242–250, 1969.

186. *Hoffman, S., et al.:*
Demineralization studies of fluoride-treated enamel using scanning electron microscopy. J. Dent. Res. 48: 1296–1301, 1969.

187. *Hoffman, S., McEwan, W. S., and Drew, C. M.:*
Scanning electron microscope studies of EDTA-treated enamel. J. Dent. Res. 48: 1234–1242, 1969.

188. *Hoffman, S.:*
Variations in surface resistance to enamel etching. J. Dent. Res. 51: 795–799, 1972.

189. *Hørsted, M., et al.:*
The structure of surface enamel with special reference to occlusal surfaces of primary and permanent teeth. Caries Res. 10: 287–296, 1976.

190. *Johnson, N. W.:*
Differences in the shape of human enamel crystallites after partial destruction by caries, EDTA and various acids. Arch. Oral Biol. 11: 1421–1424, 1966.

191. *Klein, H. and Knutson, J. W.:*
Studies on dental caries. XIII. Effect of ammoniacal silver nitrate on caries in the first permanent molar. JADA 29: 1420–1426, 1942.

192. *Mannerberg, F.:*
Changes in the enamel surface in cases of erosion. Arch. Oral Biol. 4: 59–62, 1961.

193. *Marshall, G. W., Olson, L. M., and Lee, C. V.:*
SEM investigation of the variability of enamel surfaces after simulated clinical acid etching for pit and fissure sealants. J. Dent. Res. 54: 1222–1231, 1975.

194. *Meckel, A. H., Griebstein, W. J., and Neal, R. J.:*
Structure of mature human dental enamel as observed by electron microscopy. Arch. Oral Biol. 10: 775–783, 1965.

195. *Mueller, B. and Tinanoff, N.:*
Enhancing retention of acid etch resin restorations in primary teeth. J. of Pedodontics. pp. 263–271, Summer 1977.

196. *Osborn, J. W.:*
The nature of the Hunter-Schreger bands in enamel. Arch. Oral Biol. 10: 929–933, 1965.

197. *Osborn, J. W.:*
Directions and interrelationship of prisms in cuspal and cervical enamel of human teeth. J. Dent. Res. 47: 395–406, 1968.

198. *Poole, D. F. G. and Brooks, A. W.:*
The arrangement of crystallites in enamel prisms. Arch. Oral Biol. 5: 14–26, 1961.

199. *Poole, D. F. G. and Johnsin, N. W.:*
The effects of different demineralizing agents on human enamel surfaces studied by scanning electron microscopy. Arch. Oral Biol. 12: 1621–1634, 1967.

200. *Raadal, M.:*
Mikrotensjon av plastfyllingsmaterialer pa syreetset emalje. Den Norske Tannlaegeforenings Tidende 85: 404–413, 1975.

201. *Retief, D. H.:*
Effect of conditioning the enamel surface with phosphoric acid. J. Dent. Res. 52: 333–341, 1973.

202. *Ripa, L. W., Gwinnett, A. J., and Buonocore, M. G.:*
The "prismless" outer layer of deciduous and permanent enamel. Arch. Oral Biol. 11: 41–48, 1966.

203. *Sharpe, A. N.:*
Influence of the crystal orientation in human enamel on its reactivity to acid as shown by high resolution microradiography. Arch. Oral Biol. 12: 583–591, 1967.

204. *Silverstone, L. M.:*
The primary translucent zone of enamel caries and of artifical caries-like lesions. Brit. Dent. J. 120: 461–471, 1966.

205. *Silverstone, L. M., et al.:*
Variation in the pattern of acid etching of human dental enamel examined by scanning electron microscopy. Caries Res. 9: 373–387, 1975.

206. *Silverstone, L. M.:*
Fissure sealants: The susceptibility to dissolution of acid-etched and subsequently abraded enamel. Caries Res. 11: 46–51, 1977.

207. *Swanson, L. T. and Beck, J. F.:*
Factors affecting bonding to human enamel with special reference to a plastic adhesive. JADA 61: 581–586, 1960.

208. *Swartz, M. L. and Phillips, R. W.:*
A method of measuring the adhesive characteristics of dental cement. JADA 50: 172–177, 1955.

209. *Wei, S. H. Y.:*
Remineralization of enamel and dentin—a review. J. Dent. Child. 34: 444–451, 1967.

Miscellaneous:

210. *Andreasen, J. O.:*
Traumatic injuries of the teeth. Munksgard, Copenhagen, Denmark, 1972.

211. *Arana, E. M.:*
Clinical observations of enamel after acid-etch procedure. JADA 89: 1103, 1974.

212. *Arnold, F. A., Jr., et al.:*
Effect of fluoridated public water supplies on dental caries prevalence, Tenth year of the Grand Rapids-Muskegon study. Public Health 71: 652–658, 1956.

213. *Asmussen, E.:*
Penetration of restorative resins into acid etched enamel. IADR abstract no. 349, February, 1977.

214. *Ast, D. B., et al.:*
Newburgh-Kingston caries-fluorine study XIV. Combined clinical and roentgenographic dental findings after ten years of fluoride experience. JADA 52: 314–325, 1956.

215. *Backer Dirks, O.:*
Longitudinal dental caries study in children 9–15 years of age. Arch. Oral Biol. 6: 94–108, 1961.

216. *Baumhammers, A.:*
Temporary and semi-permanent splinting. Charles C. Thomas, Publisher, Springfield, Illinois, 1971.

217. *Bhaskar, S. N. and Frisch, J.:*
Use of cyanoacrylate adhesives in dentistry. JADA 77: 831–837, 1968.

218. *Bodecker, C. F.:*
Enamel fissure eradication. NYSJD 30: April 64, 149–154.

219. *Bodecker, C. F.:*
Dental caries immunization without fillings. NYSDJ 30: October 6, 337.

220. *Buonocore, M. G.:*
A simple method of increasing the adhesion of acrylic filling materials to enamel surfaces. J. Dent. Res. 34: 849–853, 1955.

221. *Buonocore, M. G.:*
Principles of adhesive retention and adhesive restorative materials. JADA 67: 382–390, 1963.

222. *Cadwell, D. E. and Johannessen, B.:*
Adhesion of restorative materials to teeth. J. Dent. Res. 50: 1517–1525, 1971.

223. *Christensen, G. J.:*
Acid etching of teeth–current status. J. of Pedodontics, pp. 187–197, Spring 1977.

224. *Cohl, M. L., Green, L. J. and Eick, J. D.:*
Bonding of clear plastic orthodontic brackets using an ultraviolet sensitive adhesive. Am. J. Orthod. 62: 400–411, 1972.

225. *Compton, F. H., Beagrie, G. S., and Chernecky, R.:*
Strength determination of periodontal splint fabricated from acid-etched retained materials. J. Periodontol. pp. 418–420, July 1977.

226. *Conway, J. C. and Baumhammers, A.:*
Scanning electron microscopic examination of surfaces and margins of restorations. J. Prosthet. Dent. 27: 622–631, 1972.

227. *Dogon, I. L.:*
Studies demonstrating the need for an intermediary resin of low viscosity for the acid etch technique. Proceedings of an International Symposium on the Acid Etch Technique. *Silverstone, L. M. and Dogon, I. L.* (Eds.) North Central Publishing Co., St. Paul, Minnesota, pp. 100–118, 1975.

228. *Dreyer Jorgensen, K. D.:*
The adaptation of composite and non-composite resins to acid etched enamel surfaces. Proceedings of an International Symposium on the Acid Etch Technique. *Silverstone, L. M. and Dogon, I. L.* (Eds.) North Central Publishing Co., St. Paul, Minnesota, pp. 93–99, 1975.

229. *Eick, J. D., et al.:*
Scanning electron microscopy of cut tooth surfaces and identification of debris by use of the electron microprobe. J. Dent. Res. 49: 1359–1368, 1970.

230. *Eick, J. D., et al.:*
Surface topography: Its influence on wetting and adhesion in a dental adhesive system. J. Dent. Res. 51: 780–788, 1972.

231. *Faunce, F. R. and Myers, D. R.:*
Laminate veneer restoration of permanent incisors. JADA 93: 790–792, 1976.

232. *Forsten, L.:*
Effect of different factors on the marginal seal of composites. IADR abstract no. 427, February, 1977.

233. *Garmen, T. A., et al.:*
A comparison of glazing materials for composite materials. JADA 95: 950–956, 1977.

234. *Gerould, C. H.:*
Electron microscope study of the mechanism of fluorine deposition in teeth. 1945.

235. *Gray, J. A., et al.:*
Electron microscopic observations of the differences in the effects of stannous fluoride and sodium fluoride on dental enamel. J. Dent. Res. 37: 638–648, 1958.

236. *Hennon, D. K. Stookey, G. K., and Muhler, J. C.:*
Prevalence and distribution of dental caries in preschool children. JADA 79: 1405–1414, 1969.

237. *Huxley, H. G.:*
The histology of rat molar tooth fissure plaque. Arch. Oral Biol. 16: 1311–1328, 1971.

238. *Hyatt, T. P.:*
Prophylactic Odontotomy: The cutting into the tooth for the prevention of disease. Dental Cosmos, pp. 234–241, 1923.

239. *Hyatt, T. P.:*
Some further considerations of the possibilities of preventive measures for the prevention of the entrance of caries into first and second permanent molars and second premolars through occlusal pits and fissures. Dental Cosmos, pp. 623–626, 1923.

240. *Jackson, D.:*
Controlled clinical trials and caries prevention. Brit. Dent. J., 425–429, 1974.

241. *Johnson, L. N.:*
Phase discrimination using scanning electron microscopy techniques. J. Dent. Res. 51: 789–794, 1972.

242. *Kurz, C.:*
A rapid indirect method for direct bonding of brackets. Dental Survey, pp. 32–34, April 1977.

243. *Lambert, P. M., Moore, D. L., and Elletson, H. H.:*
In vitro retentive strength of fixed bridges constructed with acrylic pontics and an ultraviolet-light-polymerized resin. JADA 92: 740–743, 1976.

244. *Laswell, H. R., Welk, D. A., and Regenos. J. W.:*
Attachment of resin restorations to acid pretreated enamel. JADA 82: 558–563, 1971.

245. *Lee, B. D., Phillips, R. W., and Swartz, M. L.:*
The influence of phosphoric acid etching on retention of acrylic resin to bovine enamel. JADA 82: 1381–1386, 1971.

246. *Lee, H. L., Jr., Swartz, M. L., and Culp, G.:*
Static load testing of dental adhesives. J. Dent. Res. 48: 211–216, 1969.

247. *Mohammed, H., Schoen, F. J., and Burrell, E. R.:*
A simple comparative adhesion test method for composite resins. IADR abstract no. 350, February, 1977.

248. *Mouradian, W. F., Graham, D., and Fernald, L.:*
A new approach to treatment of tetracycline stained teeth: report of a case. J. Dent. Child. pp. 35–37, 1976.

249. *Nelson, S. R., Till, M. J., and Hinding, J. H.:*
Comparison of materials and methods used in acid etch restorative procedures. JADA 89: 1123–1126, 1974.

250. *Newman, C. V. and Facq, J. M.:*
The effects of adhesive systems on tooth surfaces. Am. J. Orthodont. 51: 67–75, 1971.

251. *Pameijer, C. H. and Stallard, R. E.:*
Application of replica techniques for use with scanning electron microscopes in dental research. J. Dent. Res. 51: 672, 1972.

252. *Retief, D. H., Dreyer, C. J., and Gavron, G.:*
Direct bonding of orthodontic attachments to teeth by means of an epoxy resin adhesive. Am. J. Orthod. 58: 21–40, 1970.

253. *Pameijer, C. H. and Stallard, R. E.:*
A pressureless replica technique for use with the scanning electron microscope. J. Dent. Res. 51: 1680, 1972.

254. *Pameijer, C. H. and Stallard, R. E.:*
Three replica techniques for biological specimen preparation. Scanning electron microscopy/1973 Part III. Proceedings of the Workshop on Scanning Electron Microscopy in Pathology, Chicago, Illinois, April 1973.

255. *Powers, J. M., Allen, L. J., and Craig, R. G.:*
Two-body abrasion of commercial and experimental restorative and coating resins and an amalgam. JADA 89: 1118–1122, 1974.

256. *Scott, D. B., and Wyckoff, R. W. G.:*
Studies of tooth surface structure by optical and electron microscopy. JADA 39: 275–282, 1949.

257. *Senzamici, N. P.:*
Emergency fixation of traumatized anterior teeth using autopolymerizing acrylic resin. J. of Pedodontics, pp. 255–260, Spring 1977.

258. *Scheer, B. and Silverstone, L. M.:*
Replacement of missing anterior teeth by etch retained bridges. J. of Int. Ass. of Dent. for Child. 6: 17–19, 1975.

259. *Silverstone, L. M.:*
The histopathology of early approximal caries in the enamel of primary teeth. J. Dent. Child., May–June 1970.

260. *Silverstone, L. M.:*
The histopathology of enamel lesions produced in vitro in teeth previously exposed to calcifying fluids. Caries Res. 4: 31–48, 1970.

261. *Silverstone, L. M.:*
Enamel caries: 1. Experimental demineralisation in vitro. The London Hospital Gazette, July 1971.

262. *Silverstone, L. M.:*
The effect of topical application of calcifying fluids on human dental enamel in vitro. J. of Int. Ass. of Dent. for Child. 2: 39–54, 1971.

263. *Silverstone, L. M.:*
Remineralization of human enamel in vitro. Proceedings of The Royal Society of Medicine. 65: 906–908, 1972.

264. *Silverstone, L. M.:*
Dental caries: The problem. Dental Update, pp. 19–26, May/June 1973.

265. *Silverstone, L. M.:*
Laboratory investigations on caries prevention. Int. Dent. J. 23: 405–413, 1973.

266. *Silverstone, L. M.:*
Fissure sealants: 1. Dental Update, pp. 163–170, July/August 1976.

267. *Silverstone, L. M.:*
Fissure sealants: 2. Dental Update, pp. 73–82, March/April 1977.

268. *Silverstone, L. M.:*
Remineralization phenomena. Caries Res. 11: 59–84, 1977.

269. *Simonsen, R. J.:*
Acid etch as a preventive technique in dentistry. Chapter 18, in A textbook of preventive dentistry. *Caldwell, R. C.* and *Stallard, R. E.* (Eds.). W. B. Saunders, Philadelphia, Pa. 1977.

270. *Swaine, T. J.* and *Wright, G. Z.:*
Direct bonding applied to space maintenance. J. of Dent. for Child., 6: 401–405, 1976.

271. *Tay, W. M.,* et al.:
An assessment of anterior restorations in vivo using the scanning electron microscope. Results after one year. Brit. Dent. J. 137: 463–471, 1974.

272. *Vig, P.* and *Silverstone, L. M.:*
Research Annotation: The advantages of direct bonding of orthodontic attachments to the enamel surface. J. Int. Ass. Dent. Child. 3: 19–20, 1972.

273. *Zachrisson, B. U.:*
The acid etch technique in orthodontics: clinical studies. Proceedings from an International Symposium on the Acid Etch Technique, North Central Publishing Co., St. Paul, Minnesota, pp. 265–275, 1975.

274. *Zachrisson, B. U.:*
A post-treatment evaluation of direct bonding in orthodontics. Am. J. of Orthod. 71: 173–189, 1977.

275. *Zachrisson, B. U.:*
Clinical experience with direct-bonded orthodontic retainers. Am. J. of Orthod. 71: 440–448, 1977.

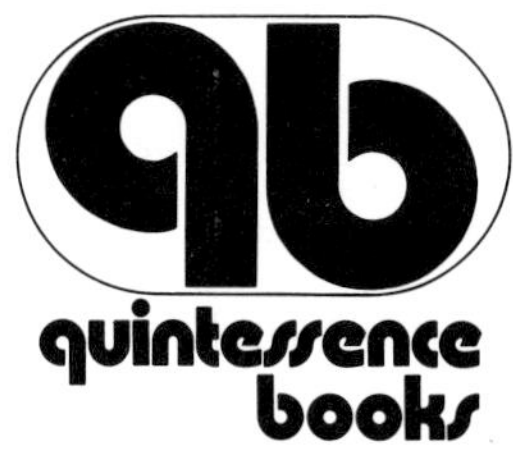

Richard W. Chaikin

Elements of Surgical Treatment in the Delivery of Periodontal Therapy

The concept of this book is to provide complete and detailed step by step photographs of various current soft tissue periodontal surgical techniques. An attempt has been made to describe the procedures in very specific detail.

Pictures were taken during the course of each phase of the procedure as well as afterwards. The detail of the technique of obtaining each particular step is thus vividly portrayed. This monograph, then, is a manual of technique with a minimum of text. By following the abundant and minutely detailed photographs, the postdoctoral student, whether in General Practice, or in a school program, may commence to refine his particular surgical technique.

Included also is a fine introductory chapter on philosophy of periodontal therapy, as well as chapters on Electrosurgery and Implantology from a periodontist's point of view.

No restorative procedure will be of value unless the supporting structures are first placed in adequate health. It, therefore, becomes the obligation of every dentist to recognize periodontal pathosis and to have it corrected for adequate biomaintainability. Since this text discusses many soft tissue problems and their corrections, it should be in the library of every dentist.

176 pp; 129 single-color and 137 multi-color illustrations; 17,5 x 24,5 cm format.
Price: $ 54.00 plus postage and 5% sales tax in Illinois/USA

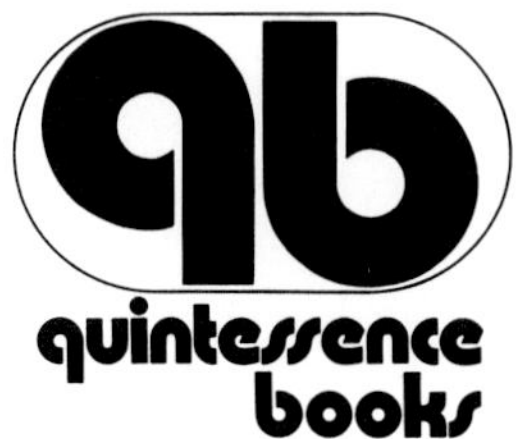

Hans R. Mühlemann

Introduction to oral preventive medicine

Many dentists use the term "preventive dentistry" synonymously with "fluoride therapy". But today, every aspect of dental practice should be considered from a preventive point of view: preventive restorative dentistry, preventive endodontics, preventive radiology, preventive periodontics and even preventive oral diagnosis. Professor Hans Mühlemann has tied prevention up in a very tidy package, originally aimed at dental students, but expanded in the English-language edition to provide a comprehensive, enlightening and often humorous review for all dentists and dental educators. The central focus is not on gray theory but rather practical observation in clinical situations.

All in all, an up-to-date look at all aspects of oral preventive medicine.

256 pages, 65 single-color illustrations, 17 x 24 cm format, washable plastic binding, price: $ 22.– plus handling and 5% sales tax in Illinois/USA.